FIRST AID

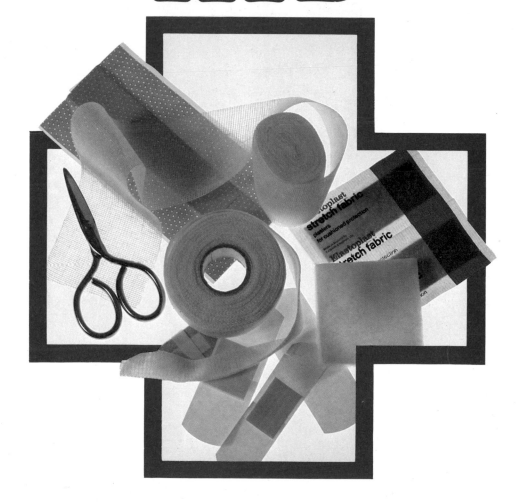

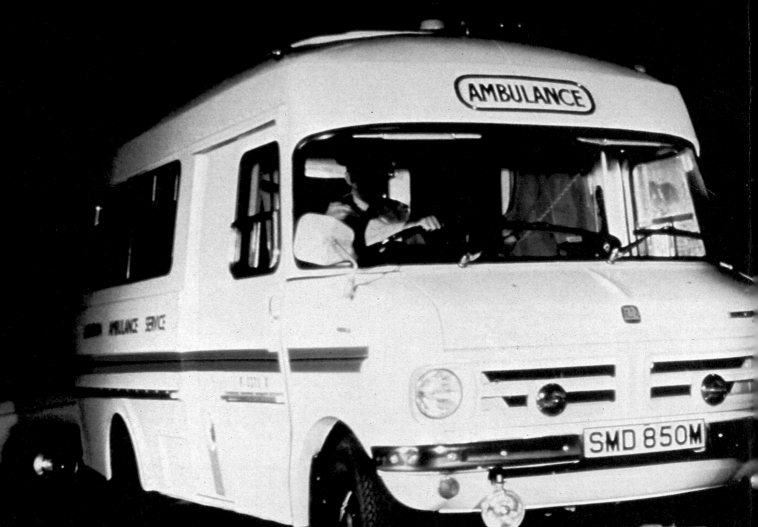

FIRST AID

ELIZABETH FENWICK

CONSULTANTS
DR PETER FENWICK
THE BRITISH RED CROSS SOCIETY

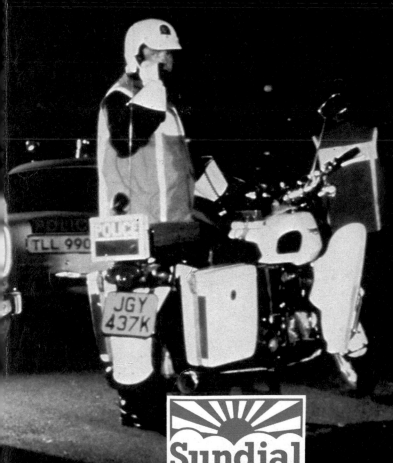

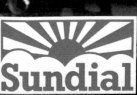

Sundial

FOREWORD

There is a natural tendency to regard First Aid as a set of procedures which are administered and received by other people. All too often it is neither known nor appreciated that more people die each day from accidents occurring in the privacy of the home than are killed either on the roads or at work.

The object of this clear and readable book is not only to make the reader more fully aware of the risk areas within the home and suggest precautionary measures but also to provide a source of reference for dealing with everyday minor accidents. However, if you should be faced with a major crisis or accident, knowing the correct emergency procedure is vital. Your prompt action could save a life. It is too late wishing you knew what to do when one of the family is lying in a crumpled, bleeding heap at the foot of the stairs while you stand helplessly by.

If, by reading this book, you or members of your family are stimulated into taking a deeper interest in First Aid, as I hope will happen, do not hestitate to put your name down for a short practical course at your nearest Red Cross Centre.

John Gray, CB MB FFCM
Chief Medical Officer BRCS

CONTENTS

ACCIDENTS WILL HAPPEN

This well known saying is probably on the lips of thousands of people every day and, alas, it is frighteningly true! We read daily of accidents on our roads, in industry and on our farms. We do not read so frequently about the accidents which occur in the 'safety' of our own homes.

Legislation exists to protect our health and safety at work, in our schools, in restaurants, public parks and on the highways and yet, 'accidents will happen'.

The degree to which we and our families are protected at home depends very much upon how aware we are of the dangers inherent in everyday activities and the special vulnerability of some members of the family to those dangers. Indeed since statistics show that almost one third of all accidents occurs behind the safety of our own front doors we are perhaps not as careful as we might be. The two age-groups in any family who are most vulnerable to accidents are undoubtedly small children and the elderly; both these groups need special protection, although anyone can have 'accidents' at any time.

During childhood and adolescence, it would seem that boys have a higher accident rate than girls. This may be because they are naturally more adventurous than girls, although that is debatable; it may simply be that parents are less restrictive and protective towards their sons than towards their daughters.

In adulthood, women seem more prone to accidents than men, although generally these are less serious accidents. We are all more accident-prone when we are tired, preoccupied, angry, upset or have drunk too much or when we are trying to do too many things at once. A woman is more likely to have accidents before or during her monthly period.

At all these times the edge is likely to be off our efficiency, and our attention is likely to lapse. And this of course is the moment when the knife will slip, we'll walk into the edge of the door, or drive straight into the back of the car in front. If you *know* you are in a fragile emotional state for any reason be extra careful, or at least think twice about doing anything potentially dangerous, whether it is driving a car, using complicated machinery or chopping up onions with a sharp knife.

In old age we all become more frail. The failing of our senses, sight, hearing, even smell will impair our ability to see obstacles in our path, hear a car or motorcycle behind us or smell burning or leaking gas. We may misread the labels on medicine bottles and our memories may also dim slightly, making us absent-minded. Once again this can lead to accidents. Our bodies are also less able to cope with extremes of temperature and we are particularly vulnerable to cold. As our joints stiffen we are more likely to lose our balance and fall over, and our bones will be far more brittle and subject to fracture. The elderly, then, need extra special care and protection even at home.

What are the hazards that make our homes so dangerous? There are some of which we are all aware, others may be less obvious and it will be these that may eventually trip us up . . . or burn us, or cause serious injury to others. So the watch word of home safety might be another well known saying, 'Prevention is better than cure'.

Right: Accidents are not always caused by excessive speed or by taking foolish risks. Whether you are a motorist, cyclist or pedestrian, a moment's inattention may be enough to cause a nasty accident.

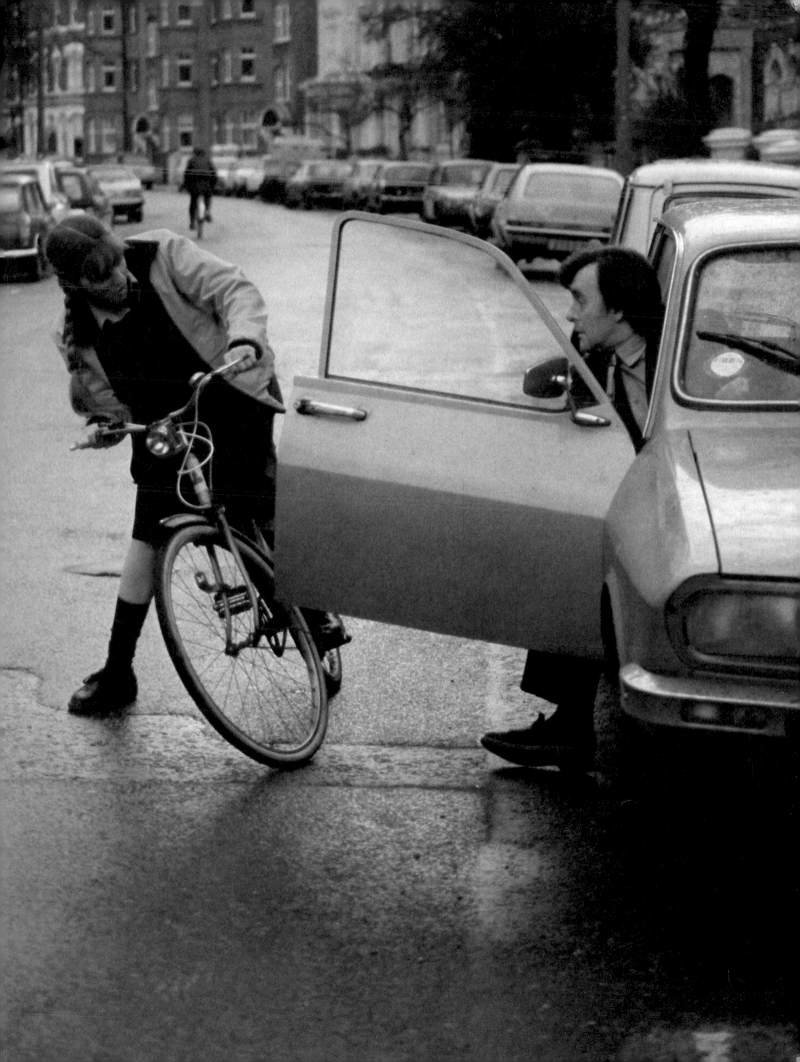

HAZARDS IN THE HOME

Because we all take our own surroundings so much for granted it is difficult for us to look at them critically enough to spot possible sources of danger. The simple check lists on the following pages are designed to help any family to pinpoint potential hazards in the home and to take the necessary action to prevent accidents in the future. No home can ever be entirely risk free, indeed life would be hardly worth living if our homes were hermetically sealed against all germs and danger. Most adults are able to cope with the risks of everyday living, but this is no reason why life should not be made easier by the removal of obvious danger and indeed most of us are responsible for those who are more vulnerable and who depend upon us for protection. Use this list to assess just how safe your home is. If you score 100 per cent – Congratulations! If not, take remedial action now!

Between the ages of 15 and 44 we are at our least accident-prone. Women in this age-group have many more accidents than men (because so many of them spend so much time in that dangerous place, the home), but the accidents men do have tend to be more severe. Women seem to be especially accident-prone just before and during their menstrual periods.

Fire is the major domestic hazard, and the kitchen is the main danger zone. Always keep pan handles turned inwards, so that you don't knock against them. If a pan of hot fat should catch fire, never try to take it outside – or to put the flames out with water. Put a pan lid or a thick, folded, damp towel over the blaze, or use a small domestic fire extinguisher. Many kitchen accidents (and irritating breakages) happen simply because there is not enough storage space or a large enough working surface to work efficiently. Remember that steam is even hotter than boiling water; if you fill a kettle which has just boiled dry you risk a scald from a sudden surge of steam.

Electrical appliances are another source of danger, either because they are not properly maintained – worn flexes, broken plugs or plugs not properly wired and earthed – or because they are used in a haphazardly dangerous way, by people who try to fish pieces of toast out of the toaster with a fork without switching it off, for example. Electric hedge clippers and lawn mowers should always be used with the cable looped over your shoulder to keep it safely out of the way of the blades. Don't use an electric lawn mower if the grass is wet or if it is raining. Never touch any electrical appliance if you have wet hands – water and electricity together make a potentially lethal combination. If you have an electric heater in your bathroom, it should be mounted on the wall well out of reach and operated by a pull-string switch. There should be no power points in your bathroom, except a specially insulated shaver point for an electric shaver.

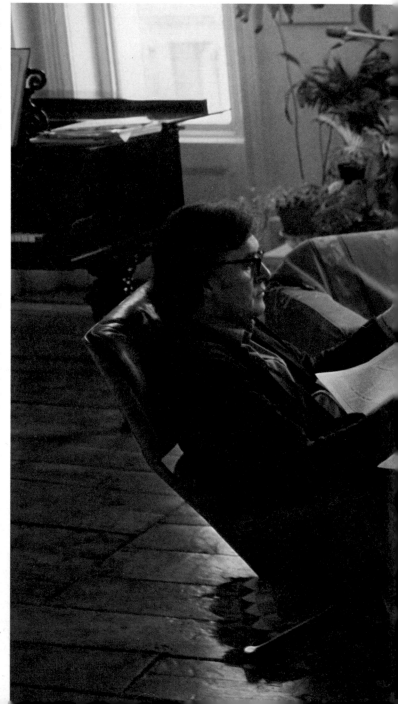

Central heating is obviously the best way to avoid fire hazards, but it isn't always possible to make this the sole form of heating.

If you have any open fires – either solid fuel, gas or electric – keep them well guarded. Resist the temptation to put mirrors above mantelpieces and above open fires to avoid the risk of clothing catching fire. Paraffin heaters are the greatest fire hazard of all. Make sure they are stable and NEVER move them while they are alight. Electric fan heaters are a safer form of bedroom heating, but whatever kind you use, make sure it stands well away from any hanging clothes, curtains or bedcovers that might be set alight.

Below: Even the happiest home can be a source of risk for the unwary. Checking your own house for potential danger-zones now is the best way to prevent accidents later.

Keeping your house in a good state of repair is a basic safety precaution. If you like to tackle home repairs yourself, use the right kind of tools for the job; not only is this much more efficient, it will be safer too than using makeshift tools. Always work in a good light, and if you are using power tools, such as sanders or saws, wear safety goggles to protect your eyes from any flying particles. When spraying paint or varnish, always wear a face mask to prevent your breathing in fine spray. Ideally, you should have, if not a proper workshop, at least a well designed bench and storage facilities so that all potentially dangerous equipment can be kept locked away out of the reach of small children. Finally, if you use any piece of complex machinery or power tool, at work or at home, concentrate on what you are doing. Don't use machinery or power equipment after drinking, or taking any drugs which might impair your general alertness (see overleaf).

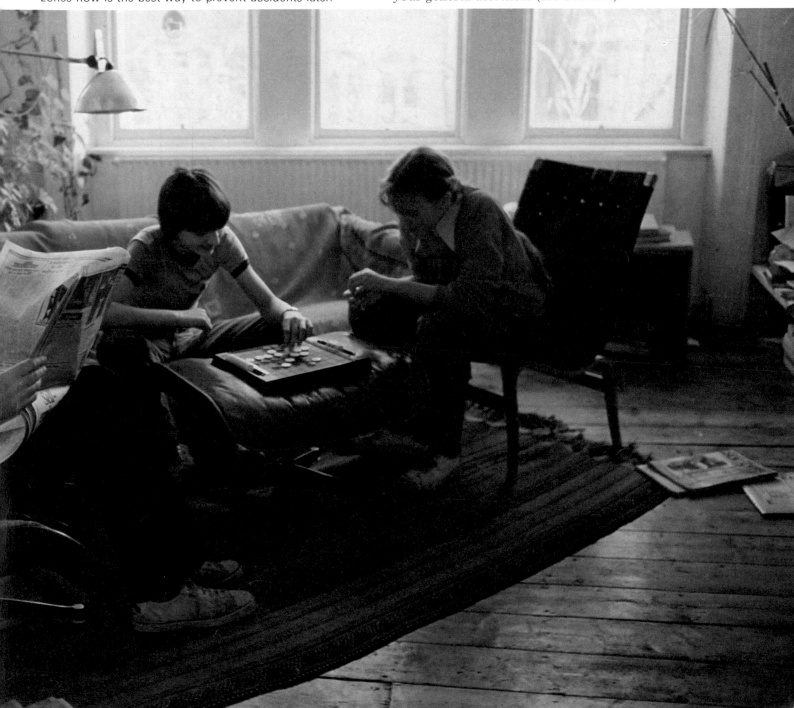

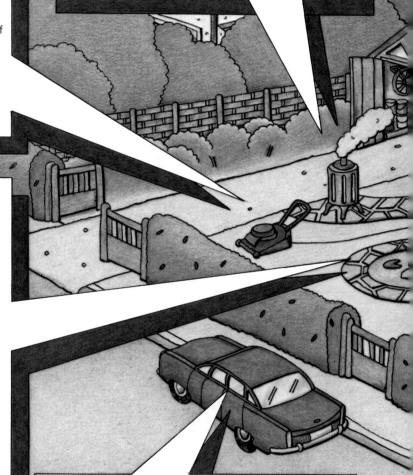

WHAT ARE YOUR CHANCES OF A FIRE?

- Is the electrical wiring in your house sound? (The Electricity Board will check this for you.)
- Are all your open fires properly guarded?
- Do you try to avoid putting mirrors over mantelpieces above open fires?
- If you have portable oil heaters, do you make sure you NEVER move them while they are still burning?
- Do you resist the temptation to warm clothes, or dry them quickly if you are in a hurry, over a heater or close to a fire?
- Do you store all inflammable liquids well away from the house?
- Do you use a proper incinerator for burning rubbish?
- If you use paraffin to get an incinerator, bonfire, or barbecue going do you always replace the cap and take the can some distance away *before* lighting the fire?
- AND do you then make sure that nobody has wandered too near before you light the fire?

HOW SAFE ARE YOUR ELECTRICAL APPLIANCES?

- Are all your electrical appliances properly wired and earthed?
- Do you check the plugs connected to your electrical appliances from time to time to make sure they are not damaged in any way?
- Do you regularly check your electric flexes for wear?
- If you have a bathroom heater, is it mounted securely on the wall, AND does it have a pull-string switch?
- If you use an electric shaver in the bathroom, do you have a specially insulated shaver point?
- Do you know that any other power outlet in the bathroom is illegal?
- Do you always switch off and unplug electrical appliances when mending or adjusting them?
- Do you have enough power points, so that you need not overload them?
- Do you know that you should never remove the back of a television set, even when it is unplugged?
- Do you switch off the television set and remove the plug from the mains each night?
- Do you always follow the instructions on your electric blanket and have it properly and regularly serviced?
- Do you use your electric lawn mower only when the grass is dry?

HOW SAFE IS YOUR GARDEN?

- Do you put away all garden implements after using them?
- Are all your garden paths and steps in good repair?
- Is your guttering in good condition?
- Are all your roof slates secure and your chimney stack in good repair?
- If you have a radio or TV aerial located on the roof of the house, is it firmly fixed?
- Do you keep all fertilizers, pesticides, weed-killers, etc. safely locked up?
- If you have a rotary mower, do you always wear strong boots or shoes when using it?
- When cutting the lawn with a power mower, do you always remove any stones from the lawn before you start?
- Do you always switch off the motor before leaving the mower unattended?
- If you are using electric shears, do you always trail the cable over the shoulder furthest from the cutting edge?
- If you have an ornamental pool and young children, is your pool fenced off or drained?
- Is your garden water butt covered?
- When staking flowers with bamboo canes, do you always make sure the stakes are at least four feet high and clearly visible, so that no-one is likely to bend over and pierce himself in the eye?
- Do you use plastic rather than glass for cold frames and cloches?

ARE YOU SAFE IN CHARGE OF A CAR?

- Do you have your car serviced regularly?
- Do you have wing mirrors fitted . . . and do you use them?
- Do you always fasten your seat-belts?
- Do you take the alcohol limits seriously?

ARE YOU A SAFE HANDY-MAN?
- Do you try always to work in a good light?
- Do you use the right tools for the job?
- Do you wear safety goggles when using sanders, saws or wire brushes?
- Do you wear a face mask if you have to spray paint, varnish or chemicals?
- Do you own an adequate, stable step-ladder?
- When using an extension ladder do you always check that it is in good repair, placed on firm, even ground and securely fastened?

HOUSEKEEPING HAZARDS
- If you have large plate-glass windows or doors are you careful not to keep them *so* clean that they are virtually invisible?
- If you have polished floors do you use a non-slip polish—and put a strip of non-slip backing on to the backs of all loose rugs?
- Do you have adequate lighting on your stairs?
- Are your carpets and other floor coverings in reasonable condition, with no holes or turned up edges to act as trip-wires?

HOW SAFE IS YOUR KITCHEN?
Women have more trivial domestic accidents than men do simply because they tend to spend much more time in the kitchen, which can be the most dangerous place in the house.
- When you are cooking, do you turn your pan handles inwards?
- Do you lift the lids of boiling pans from the far side to avoid scalding yourself?
- If your frying or chip pan catches fire, do you know how to put it out?
- Do you own and use a proper oven-cloth or gloves?
- Is your cooker positioned well away from any curtains?
- Is your kitchen floor non-slip, even when it is wet?
- Have you got enough storage space and adequate working surfaces?
- Do you realize that you ought to discard chipped or cracked crockery (even if you can't bring yourself to do it)?
- Do you have a gas, foam or dry-powder fire-extinguisher in your kitchen?

ARE YOU RUNNING A RISK OF ACCIDENTAL POISONING?
- If you reheat previously cooked food, do you make sure it is heated through very thoroughly?
- If you are preparing frozen chicken, do you let it thaw properly before you cook it?
- Do you keep cream and milk products cool and covered, especially in hot weather?
- Do you keep all medicines labelled correctly, and throw them away when an illness is over?
- Are you careful never to store poisonous substances in innocent-looking containers, for example white spirit in a gin bottle?
- Do you know that if you pour both bleach AND a proprietary lavatory cleanser down a sink or a lavatory, poisonous chlorine gas is given off?

KEEPING YOUR CHILD SAFE

During infancy it is relatively easy to keep your child safe. His environment is one that you create for him, and most of the potential dangers that might face him are ones that *you* can foresee and therefore avoid. But once he starts to move about, even a little, things are quite different. About a quarter of all home-based accidents involve children under the age of four. The home that was safe for *you* will not be safe for your child – and the one that is safe for him at six months may be a death-trap six months later. One of the difficulties of keeping a child safe is to keep one jump ahead of him. The day you decide that he'll need safety straps in his high-chair pretty soon will be the day he'll discover how to climb – and fall out of it. So put the fire-guards around the fires before he learns to crawl, and fix the safety-gate to the stairs before he tries to climb them. You cannot, and should not, stop a child exploring, but it is up to you to make his world safe for him to do so. The safer your home, the fewer the risks he will run, but most children are so enterprising and most adults so fallible that there is probably no such thing as a risk-free environment for a child under three years old, unless it is a padded cell. Most of the time he likes to be where you are, which makes it relatively easy to keep a watchful eye on him. But from the time he can move around under his own steam until the time he has learned a little common sense and forethought (always later than you would think), one simple rule holds good: if you don't know where he is, he is probably up to no good and at risk from something you have overlooked. Below are some of the special risks a very young child can run, and ways you can prevent them.

SUFFOCATION, CHOKING AND DROWNING

Suffocation and choking are by far the greatest causes of accidental death in children under five. The smaller and more helpless the child, the more vulnerable he is.

Anything that blocks your child's airway will suffocate him. Treat plastic bags like a potential source of poison. Lock them away if you keep them, tear them up before you throw them in a waste paper basket. Cot mattresses may be sold wrapped in a protective cover. Never leave this on, and never use a thin plastic sheet as a waterproof cover for a cot or pram mattress. If you want to use a pillow for a small baby, make sure it is hard, so that his face cannot sink into it. Babies do not really need pillows at all and are better, and *safer*, sleep-ing flat. If you want to prop your baby up, put the pillow under the head of his mattress. Put your baby to sleep on his tummy when he is tiny, so that if he brings back any milk he is unlikely to choke. Never leave a baby alone with a feeding bottle propped up in his mouth – he could easily choke. Any small object is a potential danger to a baby. Until he is at least a year old he will put anything and everything into his mouth. Don't stop him doing this – it isn't possible, and anyway this is the natural way for a baby of this age to explore his surroundings. But do make sure that the objects available to him are safe, smooth, and too large for him to swallow or choke on.

If you have a deep freeze, keep it locked. An older, inquisitive child could climb in and be trapped.

When you are bathing your child, keep a firm hold on him all the time until he can sit up quite safely on his own in the bath, and even then don't leave him in the bathroom alone until he is at least two and a half to three years old. Garden waterbutts and pools should be covered until children are old enough to be safe with them. Empty garden paddling pools after use – a child can drown in even a small depth of water.

The best safety measure of all is to teach your child to swim at the earliest possible age. When you are at the seaside, always keep inflatable water toys on a line, and always wear life jackets if you are out in a boat. Never let your child play near water unless he has an adult with him – and that doesn't mean just dozing on the bank. Keep sandpits shallow, so that your child cannot bury himself or another child.

POISONING

About a quarter of a million toxic products are on general sale and the chances are high that you will have a number of these around your home. No toddler is a gourmet – he will taste indiscriminately anything he comes across, or have an experimental swig at any bottle left within his reach.

Most accidental poisoning is by medicine – a single adult dose may kill a child, and many medicines are sold in a form that looks dangerously like sweets. Make sure that your medicine cabinet is inaccessible AND securely fastened with a safety lock. Having done this, KEEP YOUR MEDICINES IN IT. It is very easy to leave the aspirin or the sleeping tablets by the bed, or to keep

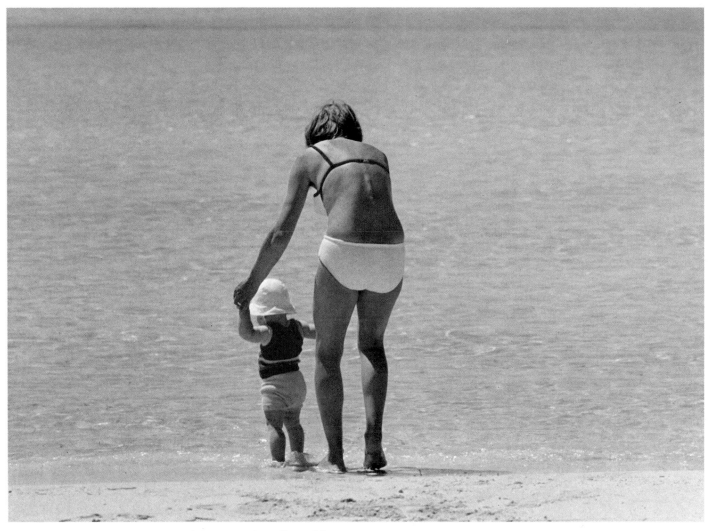

pills you have to take regularly in your handbag. If you do have to carry tablets around with you, keep them in a child-proof container.

Your child will probably come to no harm if he eats your lipstick or eye shadow, but some cosmetics, nail varnish or remover, or hair sprays, may be poisonous. Play safe and keep them all out of reach.

Lock away all cleaning materials, liquids, soaps, detergents, bleaches. Assume that they are all harmful, and indeed most of them are. The kitchen is as potentially dangerous as the medicine cabinet. Keep workshops and garden sheds locked too. Paint, paint-strippers, thinners, removers and any other chemicals should be inaccessible. So too should all insecticides, weed killers, fertilizers, etc.

Less obvious perhaps, but particularly dangerous because we treat them so casually that we tend to forget they are poisonous, are alcohol, matches and tobacco.

For a bottle-fed baby, food poisoning can be a real risk. Sterilize all the equipment you use carefully – milk is an ideal breeding ground for bacteria. Never leave prepared feeds standing around at room temperature, or keep the remains of one feed for the next.

Above: Most small children love the water if they are introduced to it gradually. But however confident a child seems, don't let him play in – or even near – the water unless an adult is close by.

FALLS

Most infant falls are caused by putting babies who can roll farther and faster than their mothers realize on to beds or table-tops to change their nappies. This kind of fall is unlikely to be serious; even so, the middle of a wide soft bed, or a rug on the floor, is the safest place to change a nappy. If you use a baby-sitter (see p. 15) don't put it on a table or other high surface unless you are nearby. Once your baby starts to crawl, use stair gates until he has learned to climb the stairs safely, but encourage him to do this as soon as he seems interested enough to try. Most children can manage to come downstairs quite safely backwards, if they are shown how, even before they can walk properly. Always use straps for high-chairs, prams and baby-sitters. Remember that windows and balconies can be dangerous for the toddler. Windows should open from the top, not the bottom, or have child-proof latches.

If you have polished floors, remember that bare feet are safe, but socks alone are not.

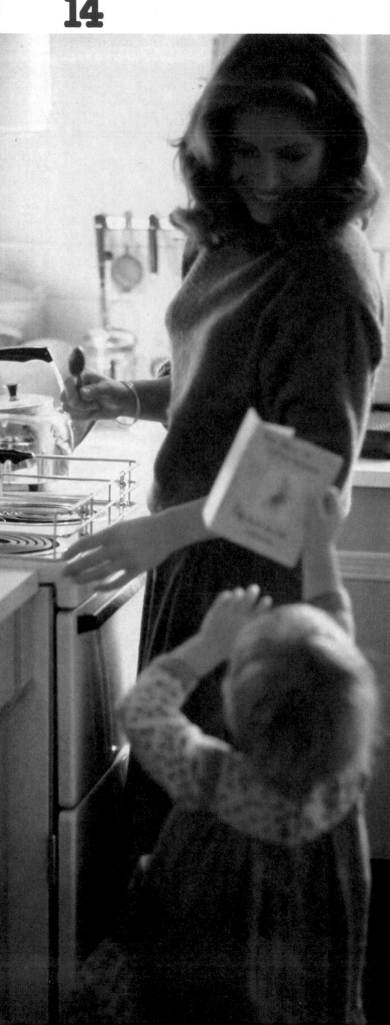

FIRES AND BURNS

While most falls in childhood are trivial, and tumbles are inevitable, burns and scalds are likely to be more serious, and should be avoidable.

For the small child, the kitchen is likely to be the most hazardous place in the house. As most small children follow their mothers around most of the time, and as most mothers spend a good deal of their time in the kitchen, your safety precautions here need to be particularly stringent.

When you are actually cooking, try to keep young children near enough to satisfy their curiosity and urge to participate, and far enough away to be out of range of splashing fat. This is the time and place for a play-pen if he will stay in it. A small child can be put in a baby-sitter, pram or baby-bouncer for at least some of the time, but there are bound to be times when your child is underfoot, whatever you are doing. Make sure that all pan handles are turned inwards, so that he cannot reach up and grab them, and have safety guards fitted to your cooker hob; these hold saucepans so that they cannot tip over. Whenever practicable use the back rings rather than the front ones, particularly if your attention is likely to be momentarily diverted.

At meal times keep hot food and drink near the centre of the table and well out of reach of young children, and don't use a table-cloth while children are still young enough to enjoy trying to pull it off.

Guard ALL FIRES, and use fixed, 'safety approved' guards. Always buy non-inflammable night-clothes for young children. Remember that electric fires, irons, cooker rings and ceramic hobs retain their heat for some time after you have switched them off.

When you bath your child, test the water carefully before you put him in. Don't run extra hot water into the bath once he is in it. If he has a hot water bottle at bed time, make sure it isn't filled with water hot enough to scald him should the bottle leak or burst.

ELECTRIC SHOCK

Block off all unused electrical sockets with special dummy plugs which can be bought for the purpose, or mask them off with heavy insulating tape. Use three-core cable and three-pin plugs so that all your electrical appliances are earthed. Keep all socket switches in the off position, so that the child has to turn two switches before anything can be turned on. Always be firm about not letting your child play with electric plugs. Even if the plugs in your home are safe, those in other people's houses may not be. Don't let a young child play with toys that are powered from the mains, and *never* let a child who is still liable to wet his bed use an electric blanket.

Left: Use the back rings of a cooker whenever possible, and turn all saucepan handles inwards. Safety guards fitted to the cooker hob will prevent saucepans tipping over.

EQUIPMENT

Make sure that all the equipment you buy is 'safety approved' by the British Safety Institute.

BABY-SITTERS: the base should be wide and sturdy, its supports should fit securely into the frame, and it must have safety-straps. For extra stability, attach rough-surfaced adhesive tape to the bottom of the frame to help prevent slipping. The manufacturers should indicate the age-range for which the chair is recommended – you will probably find that it is only safe until about six months of age.

WALKING FRAMES: for stability, the wheel base should be longer and wider than the frame. Make sure that the frame has no angles or sharp edges.

CARRY-COTS AND COTS

By the time your baby is over six months old a carry-cot on a stand is too unstable to use as a pram for him to sleep in. When you are buying a cot (or a play-pen), make sure that the rails are not more than 60 mm (2½ in) apart. Choose as deep a cot as possible – by the time your baby can pull himself upright, if the side is less than three-quarters of his height, he may easily overbalance and tip himself over the edge.

TOYS

A great many toys are unsafe, either because they are badly made or made of dangerously unsuitable materials, but most toy manufacturers try to make their products as safe as possible. It is up to you to choose toys suitable for your own child's age, and to give him a certain amount of supervision when he plays with them. Look out for, and avoid: lead paint (all painted toys and paints should be labelled 'Non Toxic'), brittle plastic, sharp edges, removable eyes, pins, staples or wires. Don't let a child under two have a pull-along toy with a string longer than 300 mm (12 in). Keep marbles well away from small children – because they are so round and smooth marbles are dangerous things for small children to choke on as they can easily become wedged across the windpipe, completely blocking off all air.

Remember that any piece of household equipment is a potential 'toy', so keep locked away any tools, sewing kits, knives, etc., that could be dangerous. As your child grows older, teach him how to use tools properly – even a four-year-old can use a saw if shown how.

CAR SAFETY

A quick survey of passing cars on any Sunday afternoon will show that an appalling number of parents let their children travel in what is the most potentially lethal position in a car – on the front passenger's knee. This is illegal in many European countries although it is still allowed in Great Britain. In any accident, the child will be first through the windscreen. A child under four should have a specially designed car seat in the back of the car. Hook-on seats with trays which are made to use as high-chairs will not do as car seats, as the child can be thrown straight out of them in a collision. Once the child is four or five he can have a properly fitted safety belt in the back seat.

Babies can travel in their carry-cot or pram top if it is safely wedged in the back seat. For extra safety, they too should be harnessed. Once your child is old enough to fiddle with the locks, make sure you have child-proof safety catches fitted to the doors at the back of the car.

Most children who are left alone in a car find it irresistible to play with the controls, however often they have been told not to. If you do have to leave them for a few moments, take out the keys, make sure the brake is on AND that the car is in gear.

When you start to back your car out of the garage at home, remember that a small child cannot be seen in your driving mirror if he is just behind the car. Pin-point his whereabouts before you start to move.

Very few children manage to get through childhood without their fingers being pinched in a car door. It is easy to do – getting in and out of cars is usually a rushed affair, once in the children are still within easy reach of the doors, and adults tend to slam the doors automatically, often without looking. Remember that the hinge side pinches just as badly as the closing side, so check both places before you close the door.

Below: A specially designed car seat, fitted in the back of a car, is essential for a small child's safety. It will give him a better view from the window too.

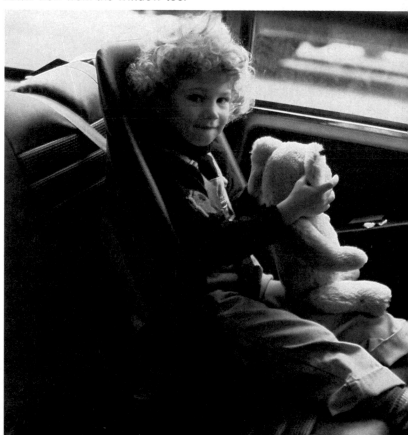

SAFETY AND THE OLDER CHILD

After the age of three the accident rate in children begins to fall, and it goes on falling throughout childhood, as the child becomes more and more able to take care of himself. But just as in infancy, it is difficult for his parents not to be always one step behind him in their awareness of what he can do. And while it is hardly possible to be too conscientious about *infant* safety, over-protectiveness of the older child can be a danger in itself. You have to allow him to stretch himself, to find his own limits, to think out for himself the risks of any particular situation. If you do all this for him he may become too timid ever to learn to do it himself. Yet he does still need your protection during these years when his sense of adventurousness outstrips his experience. The more he knows, the more experience he has, the safer he will be. It is far safer to teach him to use a penknife or a saw correctly than to forbid him to use them at all.

ROAD SAFETY

Over 50,000 children under 15 are involved in road accidents each year, and it seems to be between the ages of 5 and 9 that a child is most vulnerable. However safety conscious you make your child, and however careful you teach him to be, he will always, to some extent, be at the mercy of other people's mistakes. However, rather more accidents are caused by children running into cars than by cars running into children; you can reduce the odds of your child being involved in a road accident very considerably if you make sure that his road sense is as good as it can possibly be, and if you make absolutely sure that he is not allowed on any road at all until he *has* road sense. When this is depends partly on the road and partly on the child, but there are a few guide-lines to follow.

Until you are absolutely sure that your child can be trusted to stay on the pavement, never let him out of the front door or garden gate alone.

While he is still at the toddler stage, hold his hand or use reins (old-fashioned but more comfortable for both of you) when you are going for a walk.

Don't let a child under five try to cross *any* road alone. Once he starts going to school, map out the safest possible route to school, with the fewest roads to cross, and start walking it with him. If there are pedestrian crossings or school crossing patrols, always cross at these points. Explain to him the dangers of trying to cross between parked cars, and teach him to look both ways before crossing, keeping a special eye out for cars that might appear round corners. Walk on the right-hand side of the street, so that you are facing oncoming traffic, and keep well away from the kerb. You know your own child best, and you will know when you think he's ready to tackle this first regular journey on his own. It will probably take several months, but this is one area where you can and should be extra cautious – the dangers are too great to take any chances. If he has to make the journey in the dark, buy him a reflective arm-band to wear.

Bicycles

Until he is at least eight or nine your child is safest cycling on the pavement – although he is not legally allowed there, the police generally turn a blind eye, in the interests of safety. Before you let your child cycle on busy roads, send him on one of the cycling proficiency courses, which are usually run by the police. Your town hall or local school will probably be able to let you know whether there is one in your area.

When buying a bike make sure it is the right size:

- 510 mm (20 in) wheels for a 5–7 year old
- 610 mm (24 in) wheels for a 7–10 year old
- 660 mm (26 in) wheels for the over 10 year old.

Check the 'fit' before you buy the bike. With his foot on the lower pedal, thigh, calf and heel should form a straight line, with the knee slightly bent. Make sure his feet can reach the ground so that he can support himself when he comes to a halt. He should have to lean only slightly forward to reach the handlebars, without stretching. The seat should be parallel to the ground, or tipped slightly upward.

CHILDREN AND PLAYGROUNDS

A playground is only as safe as its equipment and the supervision given to the children using it. The fact that some 250,000 accidents happen each year to children in playgrounds is a good indication of just how far short of reasonable safety standards many playgrounds fall. Equipment is often poorly designed, inadequately maintained and badly sited. The surface on which it stands is all too often concrete, popular with local councils because it is so cheap to maintain, but potentially lethal to a falling child. There should be enough space

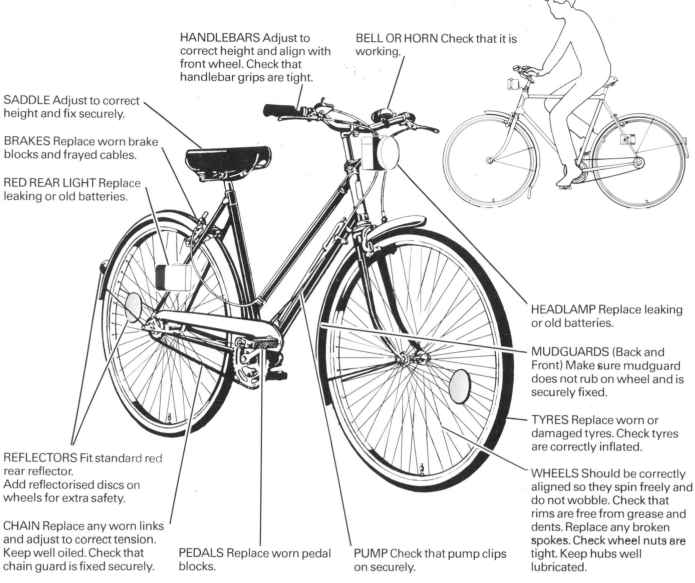

HANDLEBARS Adjust to correct height and align with front wheel. Check that handlebar grips are tight.

BELL OR HORN Check that it is working.

SADDLE Adjust to correct height and fix securely.

BRAKES Replace worn brake blocks and frayed cables.

RED REAR LIGHT Replace leaking or old batteries.

HEADLAMP Replace leaking or old batteries.

MUDGUARDS (Back and Front) Make sure mudguard does not rub on wheel and is securely fixed.

TYRES Replace worn or damaged tyres. Check tyres are correctly inflated.

REFLECTORS Fit standard red rear reflector.
Add reflectorised discs on wheels for extra safety.

WHEELS Should be correctly aligned so they spin freely and do not wobble. Check that rims are free from grease and dents. Replace any broken spokes. Check wheel nuts are tight. Keep hubs well lubricated.

CHAIN Replace any worn links and adjust to correct tension. Keep well oiled. Check that chain guard is fixed securely.

PEDALS Replace worn pedal blocks.

PUMP Check that pump clips on securely.

Above: Every child will want a bicycle sooner or later, and it is very tempting to buy one that he will 'grow into'. Don't. He'll be much safer on a bike of the right size.
Right: For bicycling at night, both children and adults should wear some kind of reflective clothing — arm bands, sash or a jacket — so that they are clearly visible to other road users.

and enough equipment for the numbers of children using the playground and if possible a 'free play' area in which older children can use bicycles, roller skates, skateboards or play ball-games. A public telephone should be somewhere near every playground, and the name and address of the nearest hospital casualty department should be clearly displayed.

Your local council is legally responsible for the safety of the playgrounds it provides. If you think that the playground your child uses does not conform to the standards you have a right to expect, contact your local Factory Inspector, listed under 'F' in the telephone directory, whose duty it is to see that councils do indeed carry out these legal responsibilities.

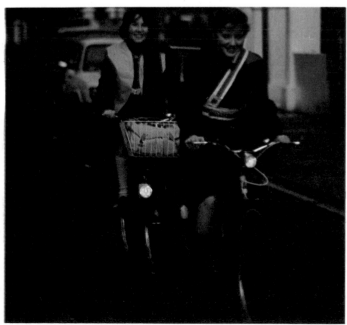

Equipment that is potentially dangerous

Three pieces of common playground equipment which have been responsible for so many accidents that they should be banned are the multi-person rocking horse, the 'ocean wave', and the plank swing.

Swings with shock-absorbent tyre seats are much safer than those with the traditional wooden seats. Swings should always be sited away from the general play area and have safety barriers in front and behind.

Slides should be no higher than 2·5 m (8 ft), and the slide section should be continuous, not assembled in panels. Sides should be built into the slide itself. Steps leading to the top of the slide should be non-slip and shallow. The sides should be panelled in, so that the child who changes his mind at the top can get safely down again. The top platform should have a solid surround or cabin structure. Safest of all are slides that are built on to an earth mound, so that the child who comes off will tumble rather than fall.

Most roundabout accidents are the result of poor installation and maintenance. Check that the timber is sound and smooth, that the roundabout turns

Below: Many playground accidents happen because the equipment is badly designed as well as poorly installed and maintained. Always supervise young children, as they can easily become frightened.

smoothly and quietly and that the underside and surrounding area is clear of litter. Because a roundabout must be clear of the ground in order to turn, there is a gap underneath it that can trap a child's feet. Teach your child to jump well clear when he is getting off and never to try to grope for anything which has rolled underneath the roundabout.

Climbing frames should be no higher than 2·5 m (8 ft), and should be built over sand. The frame itself should have no sharp projections and no open-ended metal tubes, and all joints should be secure.

A see-saw that hits the ground, or reverses its direction very sharply can dangerously jolt a child's spine. It should brake before it changes direction and the central mechanism should be safely covered; the seats and handgrips secure.

Paddling pools should be fenced in, regularly drained and chlorinated. A greater risk than lack of cleanliness is that of cut feet from pieces of broken glass or sharp broken edges in the pool lining.

A sandpit should be fenced off to prevent fouling by cats and dogs, and kept free of litter and debris. It should contain about 450 mm (18 in) of clean sand. Teach your child never to throw sand and always supervise him while he is playing. Even the best maintained playgrounds can't prevent a child getting an eyeful of sand if he steps on another child's painstaking reconstruction of Windsor Castle.

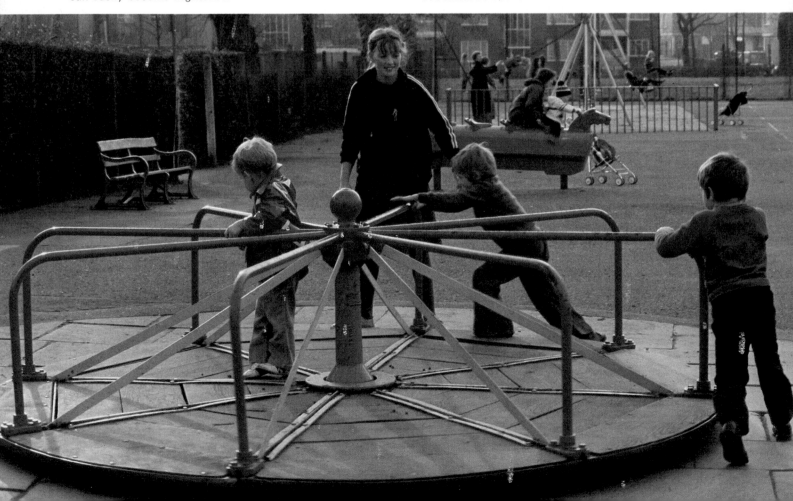

OUTDOOR ACTIVITIES

WALKING, CLIMBING AND CAVING

While you may not need expert training in order to enjoy hill-walking or mountain-scrambling you will need protective clothing, and anyone who wants to try rock-climbing, or explore caves or pot-holes should always go in the company of experts. Nearly all accidents in outdoor activities like these are caused by lack of proper preparation.

You cannot set out on a serious hill-walk with the minimal preparations you would make for a gentle ramble along country roads, with a random route and no estimated time of arrival. Always carry a large-scale Ordnance Survey map and a compass. Plot your route before you go and estimate, as far as is possible, how long it will take you. If you keep up a reasonable pace over rough ground you should be able to average about two miles per hour – but not much more. Fifteen miles is about the most you should aim to do in one day. Leave a copy of your route-plan and time-table with someone whose brief it is to start a rescue operation if you do not turn up at the appointed time (allowing a margin of a couple of hours or so for error).

If you do get lost, or injured, or have to hole up because of the weather, you will be in no real danger provided you can keep warm and dry. Seek shelter out of the wind. Make sure that your outer clothing is warm and waterproof, remembering that the weather can change quickly and the temperature drop dramatically in the hills, even in summer. Wear good strong boots which support your ankles and are roomy enough for you to wear a couple of pairs of socks, which also helps to prevent blisters.

Your rucksack should contain a survival kit: a torch and whistle, a heavy duty polythene bag which can be utilized as an emergency sleeping bag, and some high energy food, such as chocolate. You should also carry an extra sweater and socks in case you need a dry change of clothing, matches and something in which to make yourself a hot drink. A folded, waxed carton will take up very little space and when opened out and filled with water can be heated gently without catching fire. Include a fire-lighter too, unless you have many years of boy-scout experience with damp twigs behind

Right: Hill-walking is both safe and enjoyable, if you are well prepared and take the right equipment.

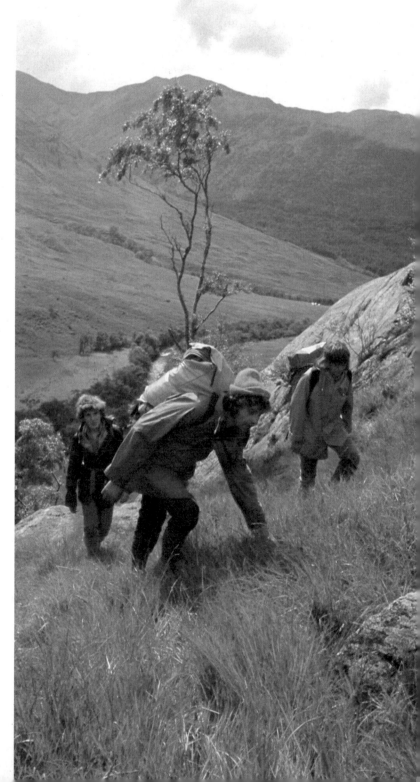

you. Carry a few adhesive dressings and a crêpe bandage too, in case of cuts, blisters or sprains.

Finally, make sure you have an accurate local weather forecast before you set out, and if you are in any doubt about the weather, don't go. Remember that if you have to be rescued by the emergency services, you are putting other lives at risk besides your own. For climbing, caving and potholing, the same rules apply – always let someone at ground level know where you are going and for approximately how long. Never go caving or potholing on your own – for maximum safety you should go in a group of about four, of whom at least one should be experienced and able to assume complete control in an emergency. Make sure you have warm, waterproof clothing and adequate equipment – this should also include emergency lighting if you are going underground. Don't attempt anything that the least experienced member of the party cannot manage easily and remember that when you are caving or pot-holing, you may need the most time, and the greatest reserves of energy, for the return journey. An important point to remember is that underground cave systems are liable to flooding, and this should be taken into account when assessing the weather before setting off.

BOATS AND WATERSPORTS

Wearing a life-jacket when you go out in a boat should be as automatic a precaution as fastening your seat-belt every time you get into a car. If you want to learn to sail on holiday, get someone who is experienced to teach you – it is asking for trouble to hire a boat you can't sail on waters you don't know. People have even come to grief in the innocent-looking 'pedalloes' which can be hired on many beaches. Only take one of these out if you are a competent swimmer and even so, stay close to the

Below: Always wear a life-jacket when sailing, however good a swimmer you are. It will keep you afloat even if you are unconscious and make you easier for rescuers to see.

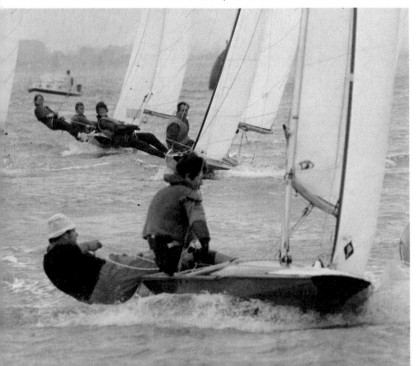

shore. Most accidents are the result of over-adventurousness; the first burst of energy takes you farther than you realize and then a sudden wind or change in the weather may make it difficult for you to get back. The same applies to swimming – always stay well within your own capabilities and unless you are a strong swimmer, swim parallel to the shore rather than away from it. Most resort beaches have notices up advising swimmers of any dangerous currents or tides, and some sort of warning system, usually red flags, if bathing is for any reason temporarily dangerous. Look out for these, and if you don't know the beach, or if it has no warning system, ask local advice about currents.

The greatest danger of sailing is not, however, drowning, but chilling. If you can swim at all and your boat capsizes, you will be able to stay afloat for quite a considerable time. *Never* leave a capsized boat to swim to the shore unless you are absolutely certain you can make it. By clinging to the boat you will be able to keep afloat much more easily as well as being a far easier target for rescuers to spot and pick up. And, just as important, by *not* attempting to swim you will be saving energy, which in turn means saving warmth. For the same reason, don't try to strip off heavy clothing if it looks as though you are obviously going to have to abandon ship. It is sensible to kick off sea-boots or Wellingtons if you are wearing them, because these would simply fill with water and weigh you down, but the thicker the sweaters or jacket you are wearing the better – however wet, they provide some insulation and will slow down the rate at which you lose heat.

WINTER SPORTS

The younger and fitter you are, the less likely you are to suffer any skiing injury. So the best safety advice to give is, start young and train before you go. Everyone falls when they are learning to ski, but the older beginner will be less supple, less relaxed and more likely to fall awkwardly and suffer breaks or sprains. However, the older skier is likely to be less reckless and know when to stop. Accidents are most likely to happen when you are tired, towards the end of the day. So stop just *before* you think you've had enough – especially at the beginning of your holiday.

Try to get some sort of pre-ski training during the three or four weeks before your holiday. Ideally you should have a few lessons on a dry ski slope, but pre-ski exercises, or even just extra walking or cycling, all of which help to strengthen the leg muscles, will make you much fitter for the slopes.

Short skis make learning to ski much easier, and safer, so if you are a novice, choose these. You will find that you will not travel so fast, and the shorter skis are much easier to control. Once you have mastered these, you can progress to a longer, more adventurous ski. Warm, waterproof clothing is particularly important. Don't try to economize by going skiing in jeans – this is especially important if it is your first attempt. You may think you will be able to keep upright and dry all

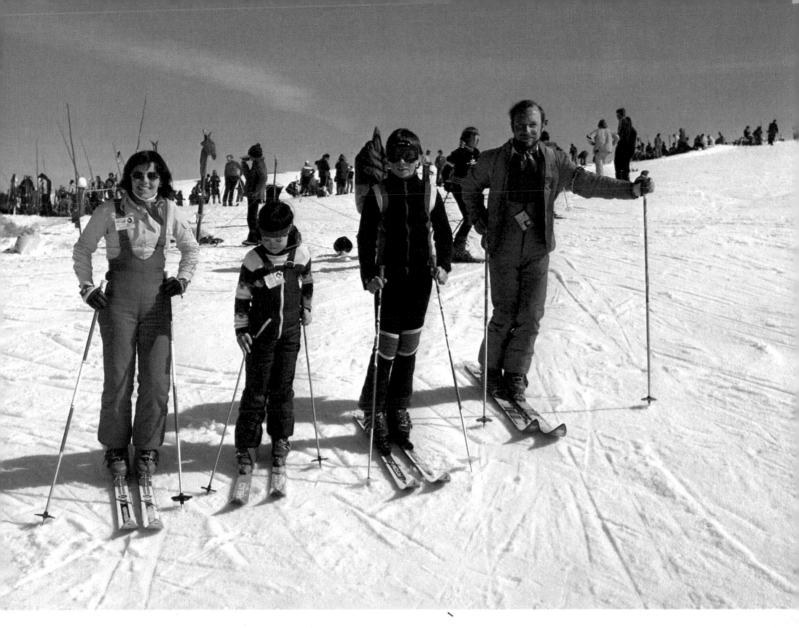

Above: When hiring skis for your holiday, always check the safety bindings and make sure the snap-release system is working properly.

day, but falls are inevitable, even for the most cautious beginner, and waterproof trousers and anorak really are essential. The high-waisted dungaree-type salopettes are comfortable, because they eliminate the gap between jersey and trousers into which cold snow can all too easily creep. You will need one or two thin jerseys, plus one thicker one, under your ski jacket or anorak. Wear two pairs of socks – and be sure that your boots are a really good fit and give your ankles plenty of support. Your skis should be fitted with safety bindings which snap open to give a quick release from your boots if you fall. Check the release mechanism each day to make sure that it is working properly. Wear waterproof (essential) mittens or gloves, and a woolly hat. Don't forget to take a suntan cream which is suitable for high altitudes and a pair of goggles to protect your eyes from the dazzle and glare of the snow. It is easy to forget the very real danger of sun (and wind) burn when you are surrounded by snow.

The beginner on the nursery slopes is unlikely to find himself at altitudes high enough to cause mountain sickness, but the more experienced skier on the higher slopes may. If you feel sick, ill, light-headed or develop a headache, go farther down the slope straight away – if the symptoms are due to high altitude, they should disappear. Mountain sickness is unlikely to occur below 3000 m (10,000 ft).

HANG GLIDING

This is an exhilarating sport, but it has its dangers, perhaps especially if you are over 40, do not fall so softly as you used to and are not really fit enough to carry an 18 kg (40 lb) glider up a steep hill. Hang gliding is a sport that will always attract people who are willing (or indeed eager) to take a few risks, and this may partly account for its relatively high accident rate. Properly learnt and practised it should be reasonably safe. In fact most hang-gliding accidents are caused through people attempting impossible manoeuvres in the wrong weather conditions – the less experienced you are, the more likely you are to do this. Whatever you do, do not casually buy a hang-glider one Saturday afternoon and then jump hopefully off the nearest cliff. Join a club where you will be taught not only how to glide as safely as possible, but which type of glider and what size would be the best for you to buy.

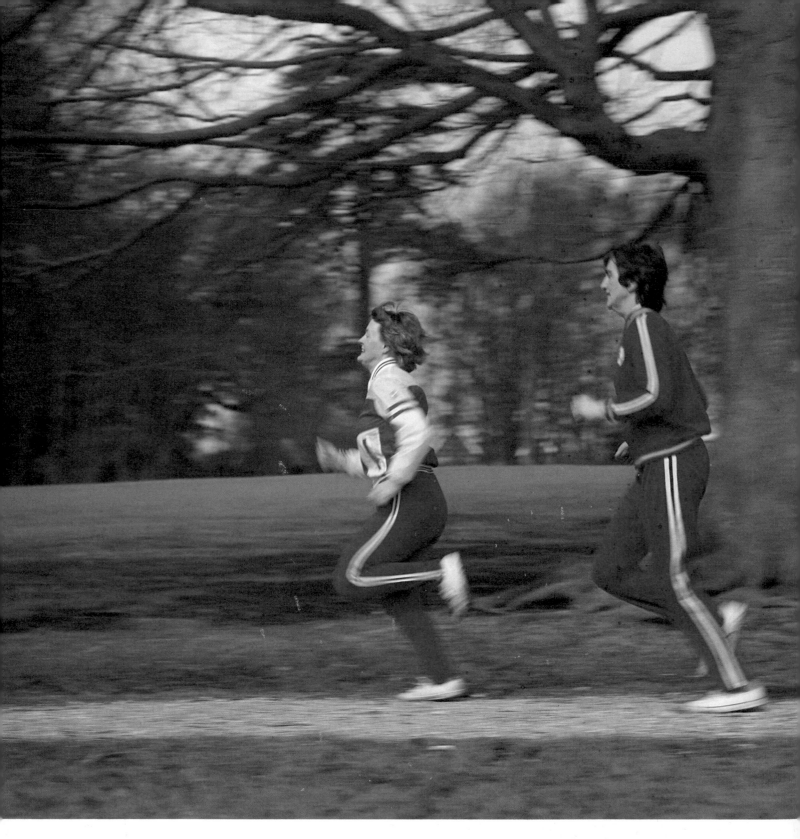

JOGGING

The knowledge that people who take regular, vigorous exercise are less likely to die of a heart attack than those who lead a sluggish or sedentary life has led to a huge increase in the number of middle-aged, track-suited city joggers. But sudden, excessive exercise taken by someone who is 40 + and unfit, especially if he is also overweight or a smoker, may actually *increase* the risk of a heart attack. Jogging, or any other form of exercise, is fine so long as you start your exercise programme slowly and build it up gradually day by day.

Above: Regular exercise makes you feel better and lowers your chances of a heart attack. Jogging is a simple way to exercise, but don't try to do too much too soon. Build up your jogging time gradually, and if you are elderly or your health is poor, consult your doctor before you start.

Don't jog just after a meal, and don't force yourself to go out if you don't really feel up to it, perhaps because you feel especially tired or generally unwell. It can be dangerous to go jogging in fog, and if you go out after dark, wear a reflective jacket or arm-bands, or at least put on light-coloured clothing so that you are easy for drivers to spot – and avoid. Wear lightweight, loose clothing, preferably with a top you can take off when you warm up. A track suit is ideal. Comfortable gym shoes are the best footwear and these should have a thick cushioned insole and no rough edges or stitches inside to rub the skin and cause blisters. Avoid choosing a shoe which is cut too high at the back as this could rub your heels.

Special precautions for elderly, unfit joggers

Start your jogging programme very gradually indeed. For your first week a brisk half-hour of WALKING each day is enough. Then, for the next two or three weeks, walk and jog alternately, jogging only for short bursts of a minute or so and stopping when you feel breathless. Your tolerance should gradually increase so that you jog more and walk less until you find that you can jog for 10–12 minutes at a stretch quite comfortably.

Don't start your jogging programme without consulting your doctor if you have suffered from:

● High blood pressure

● Heart disease

● Any chest trouble, such as bronchitis or asthma

● Arthritis or a bad back

● Or if you are convalescing from an illness or an operation.

DRIVING

For many of us motoring is a pleasure or a sport as well as just a means of transport, so it is a pity that it ranks as one of the most dangerous activities we can pursue. To make it as safe as possible, both driver and vehicle should be in good condition. You should not, for example, attempt to drive if you are drunk, drugged, angry or upset. The quantity of drink that makes us unfit to drive is probably rather smaller than most of us would like to believe. The legal limit of alcohol in the blood is 80 mg per 100 ml, which is what you would expect to reach after you have drunk 2 double whiskies (1 double whisky = 1 pint of beer or 2 standard glasses of wine), although this does vary from person to person. Many drugs affect our attention and concentration to such an extent that they make us a danger at the wheel. If your doctor prescribes such a drug he should warn you of its dangers – the tranquillizer diazepam and many anti-depressant drugs are likely to make you less alert and therefore less fit to drive. Cold cures, travel sickness pills and any drugs containing anti-histamine, such as you might take for hay fever or other allergic conditions, may also make you drowsy. Driving when you are in a highly emotional state will also make you a danger both to yourself and to anyone else on the road – the kind of internal conversations we carry on with people we are very angry with take up most of the attention that should be given to the road ahead.

Always fasten your seat-belt, and refuse to start the car until your passenger has fastened his. This should be a reflex action on even the shortest journey.

Make sure your car is kept in good condition and regularly serviced. Worn tyres are not only illegal, they are dangerous too. See that they are correctly inflated and remember that if the car is very heavily laden, particularly when you are going on holiday and possibly travelling a considerable distance, you should increase the pressure in the tyres to the recommended specification. If you do not have side mirrors on your car, have them fitted. Use them whenever you are parking, reversing, overtaking or pulling out.

Do not drive or try to use any complex machinery if you have been taking any of the following: Sleeping pills, tranquillizers, anti-depressants, antihistamines, anti-convulsants (anti-epileptic drugs), alcohol or any intoxicating narcotic or hallucinogenic drugs such as cannabis, LSD etc. Some proprietary brands of cough medicine or tonics contain either alcohol or sedative drugs, so if you regularly take one of these ask your doctor if it is safe to drive.

PROTECTING YOUR SKIN

Skin which is exposed to the sun for gradually lengthening periods will tan and the dark pigment which this produces in the skin acts as a protective barrier against the sun's rays. Dark skin tans much more easily than fair, so if you are fair or red-haired take extra care not to spend too much time in the sun, particularly on the first day or two of your holiday. It is the short, ultra-violet rays of the sun that burn. Special barrier creams are available which screen out most of the burning rays but allow the longer, tanning rays through. However, these creams are not 100 per cent effective, so don't be lulled into a false sense of security by the mere fact you are covered in sun lotion – you can still burn if you over-do the sun-bathing. Take your tanning carefully at first. Half an hour on the first day is plenty, less if you are fair-skinned or the sun is very hot. Remember that the sun is at its hottest at mid-day and can burn particularly badly if you are on or near water, because the rays are reflected off the water as well as beating down on you from above. It is easy to underestimate the power of the sun on a windy day or to forget to re-apply your screening cream after you have been swimming.

Most adults have learnt, usually through bitter experience, how much sun they can tolerate. Children have no such built-in warning system and are quite incapable of judging when they have had enough or too much. Sunburn does not hurt when it is actually happening, only hours afterwards. Neither does the skin start to redden until after the damage has been done. So keep children covered up if they spend a long time on the beach until their skins have become used to the sun. Sun hats are particularly important for children.

POISONOUS PLANTS & FUNGI

Although many of the thousands of plants and fungi native to the British Isles are edible, some are poisonous and a few can be fatal, especially if large amounts are eaten. This chart will help you identify some of the most common poisonous plants and fungi found throughout the countryside.

FUNGI

1 Death Cap
   Amanita phalloides
2 Panther Cap
   Amanita pantherina
3 Devil's Boletus
   Boletus satanas
4 Fly Agaric
   Amanita muscaria

5 Destroying Angel
   Amanita virosa
6 The Blusher
   Amanita rubescens
7 Yellow Stainer
   Agaricus xanthodermus

PLANTS

8 Mistletoe
   Viscum album
9 Hemlock
   Conium maculatum
10 Laburnum
   Laburnum anagyroides
11 Yew
   Taxus baccata
12 Monkshood
   Aconitum napellus
13 Cowbane
   Cicuta virosa
14 Larkspur
   Delphinium ambiguum
15 Thorn Apple
   Datura stramonium
16 Foxglove
   Digitalis purpurea
17 Cherry Laurel
   Prunus laurocerasus

18 Cuckoo Pint
   Arum maculatum
19 Green Hellebore
   Helleborus viridis
20 Henbane
   Hyoscyamus niger
21 Lily of the Valley
   Convallaria majalis
22 Rhododendron
   Rhododendron ponticum
23 Ivy
   Hedera helix
24 Black Bryony
   Tamus communis
25 Deadly Nightshade
   Atropa belladonna
26 Privet
   Ligustrum vulgare

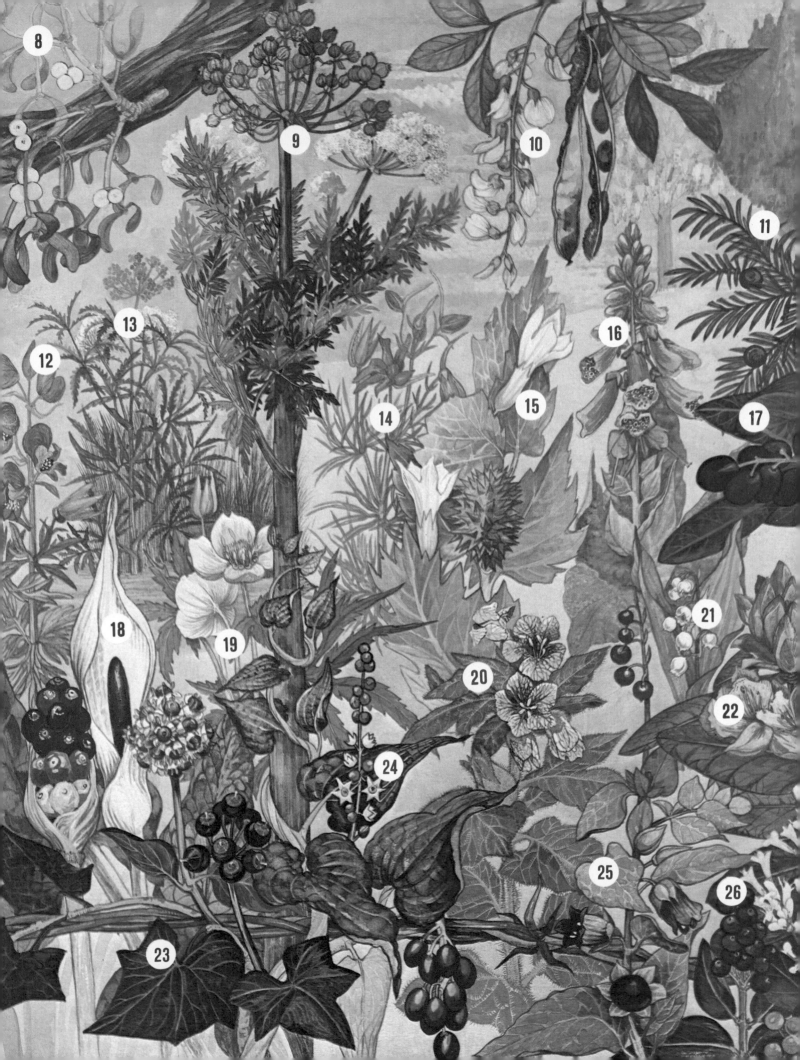

HOLIDAY TRAVEL

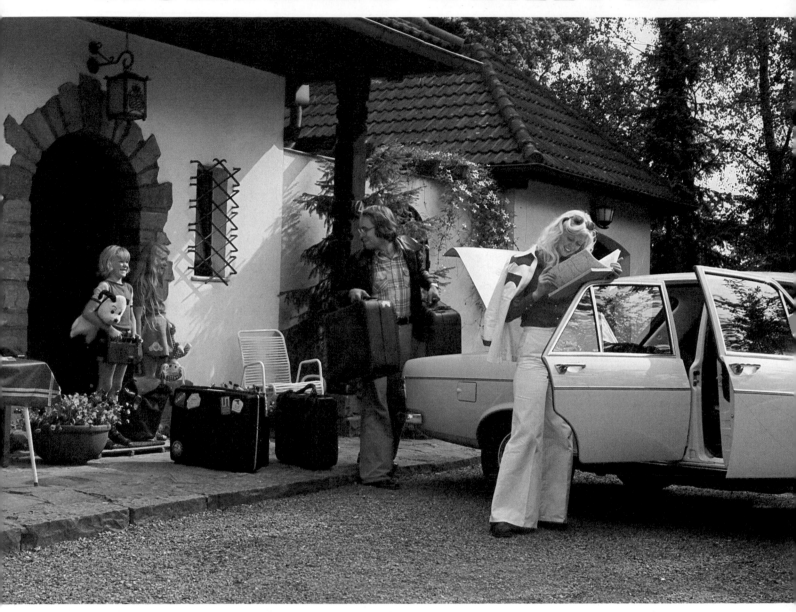

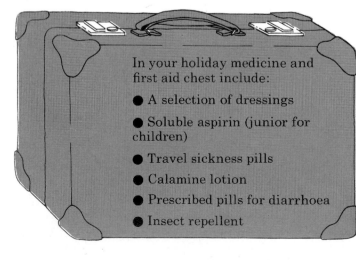

In your holiday medicine and first aid chest include:

- A selection of dressings
- Soluble aspirin (junior for children)
- Travel sickness pills
- Calamine lotion
- Prescribed pills for diarrhoea
- Insect repellent

If you are visiting a country where the water is not safe to drink, take some water sterilizing tablets (these are available from most chemists). Use these tablets if boiled water is not available for cleaning your teeth. They taste rather nasty, so if you want to drink the water, take a bottle of orange squash as well.

Avoid eating uncooked vegetables, and wash and peel fruit. Ice-cream can also cause tummy upsets, particularly in countries where the standard of hygiene is low. Unless it is purified do not have ice in your drinks, and choose bottled or fresh fruit juices, rather than squashes which need to be diluted.

If you are going somewhere very hot, take a supply of salt tablets.

IMMUNIZATIONS FOR HOLIDAYS ABROAD

The vaccination certificates required for travel abroad differ from country to country, and their requirements may vary from time to time. Check well in advance what vaccinations are needed in the countries you plan to visit. It is sometimes advisable to have protection against infectious diseases even if it is not an essential entry requirement. A rough guide is given below, but your doctor, Health Board, or the passenger immunization and medical centres of British Airways will always give you up-to-date advice about this.

Smallpox

Although smallpox has now been officially eradicated, some countries *do* still make smallpox vaccination a requirement of entry.

Plague

Immunization is advisable for visitors to the Far East.

Yellow Fever

Compulsory for most of Africa and Asia.

Cholera

Compulsory for most of Africa and Asia and advisable nearly everywhere – even in Europe.

Polio

Advisable nearly everywhere.

Hepatitis

Advisable outside Europe, especially for overlanders travelling through India.

Typhoid and Tetanus

Advisable everywhere, including Europe.

Malaria

Advisable in Africa, India, Central and South America, and the Middle and Far East. Prevention is by tablets obtainable on prescription. The usual method is to take a once-weekly dose of a drug called pyrimethamine, starting the week before you go and continuing for four weeks after your return. An alternative method is to take a daily dose of proguanil.

Left: Illness can spoil any holiday. Pack a medicine and first aid kit and, if travelling abroad, have all necessary immunizations.

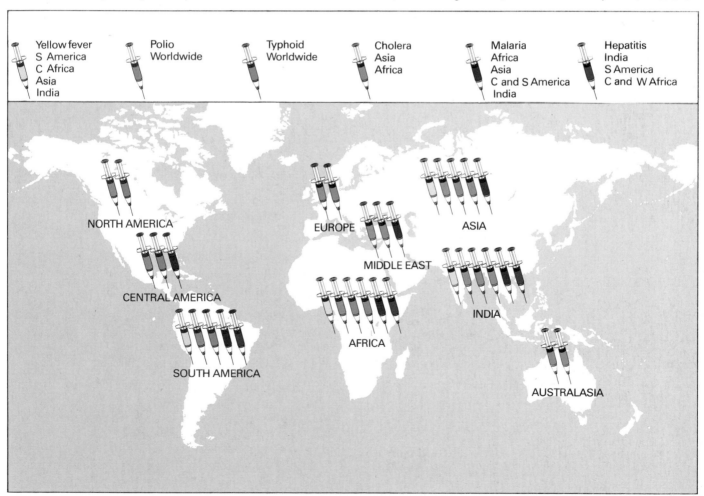

HOW TO GUARD AGAINST A
HEART ATTACK

Like any other part of the body, the heart needs oxygen and it gets it through its own blood supply – the coronary arteries. Like all other blood vessels in the body, these arteries may gradually become silted up by a fatty material called *atheroma* which becomes deposited in the lining of the arteries so that their walls become thicker and the inner canal of the artery narrower. This build-up of atheroma probably begins in childhood, although its effects are seldom noticed until middle-age, or possibly even later if you are a woman.

Once the arteries that bring blood to the heart have become narrowed (coronary artery disease), the heart may receive a perfectly adequate blood supply for most of the time, but run short if it has to work harder than usual, for example during exercise or periods of excitement or anxiety. In situations like these the supply of oxygen to the heart muscle may be insufficient for the work it has to do and it is this that results in the chest pain called *angina*. Because the arteries are not actually blocked, when the exercise or emotional stress stops, so does the pain.

While the normal lining of the arteries is very smooth, the atheromatous deposit is roughened, so that the blood, instead of flowing smoothly over it, becomes more turbulent. This makes some of the smaller blood cells, the platelets, become sticky and mass together on the roughened walls, trapping other, larger blood cells until a clot is formed which may be sizeable enough to block the artery completely, cutting off the supply to part of the heart muscle. This is what we call a *heart attack* or *coronary thrombosis*. The severity of the attack depends on where the blockage occurs. A small clot lodging in a tiny branch of an artery will deprive only a small area of heart muscle of its blood supply. This muscle will die and be replaced by inelastic scar tissue, but the heart as a whole will be able to carry on working. A first heart attack is unlikely to be severe enough to stop the heart beating altogether, but even a minor one should serve as a warning that something worse may happen unless you take action to prevent it.

Few people realize that even minimal changes in their habits and life-style could considerably improve their chances of never having a heart attack. Of these, the most important are to give up smoking, or at least to cut down the number of cigarettes you smoke, to alter your diet, and to try to lead a more tranquil life. Even if you have already suffered a heart attack, a few changes now could prevent further attacks.

A high risk candidate for a heart attack is the stocky male, aged 60 or over, with high blood pressure, who smokes 40 cigarettes a day or more. He substantially increases his chances of a heart attack if he is 12 kg (28 lb) or more overweight, takes no exercise, has a diet heavy in meat, butter, cream and eggs, and has one or more close relatives with heart disease. While not all these 'risk factors' are preventable – there is little you can do about your age, sex or the health of your relatives – a good number of them are.

THE RISK FACTORS

You are most at risk if:
● You are a man. Women are much less likely than men to have heart attacks, although after the age of 60, the risk for both sexes is virtually the same.
● Your diet contains a high proportion of animal fats – butter, cheese, cream, eggs, meat – and saturated vegetable fats such as 'hard' margarines. All these foods

de-oxygenated blood from heart to lungs

oxygenated blood from lungs to heart

de-oxygenated blood from body to heart

oxygenated blood from heart to body

Above: The human body has a 'double' circulatory system. Oxygenated blood is pumped around the body, returns to the heart and is then pumped through the lungs to be oxygenated once more.

are rich in cholesterol, from which atheroma is formed.

You are overweight.

You take little or no exercise.

You have high blood pressure (above 140/95).

You smoke. Twice as many smokers as non-smokers die of heart disease. The more you smoke, the greater the risk.

● You have one or more close relatives (parents, grandparents, brothers or sisters) with heart disease.

You are the sort of person who actually likes leading a rather stressful life: you are motivated by drive and ambition – unable to relax properly, preferring to work or play until you are exhausted.

You have diabetes. The risk of coronary artery disease is doubled for men with diabetes and is about five times as great for women.

You live in a soft water area.

WHAT YOU CAN DO TO LESSEN THE RISK OF A HEART ATTACK

1 DIET. Eat less meat – which contains a lot of fat even though you may not be able to see it – and more poultry and fish. Grill or casserole, rather than fry any meat.

Don't eat more than one egg per day.

Try to persuade yourself that you cannot tell soft, polyunsaturated margarines from butter. If you can't resist butter, try to cut down on the amount you use.

Eat less cream.

Use polyunsaturated oils rather than butter or lard for cooking. Corn, soya bean, olive, sunflower and safflower oils are all polyunsaturated. Avoid buying oils that are simply labelled 'Vegetable Oil', as these may in fact contain saturated oil.

Eat less sugar by cutting down on soft drinks and cakes, etc.

2 LOSE WEIGHT. Following the right sort of diet will probably be enough in itself to do this.

The more overweight you are, the less exercise you are likely to take, and it is this that makes fat people more at risk from coronary artery disease.

3 GIVE UP SMOKING. Try, if possible, to give up smoking altogether. If not, at least try to cut down to less than five cigarettes a day and change to a low-tar, filter tip brand. Do not inhale.

4 Start a graduated exercise programme. If you are over 35 and unfit, take it very slowly at first. Sudden and unaccustomed exercise in the middle-aged and unfit may actually *increase* the risk of a heart attack.

Walking, provided it is brisk and not just a gentle stroll, using the stairs instead of lifts – and running, rather than just walking up the stairs, are all easy ways of getting some exercise every day.

Whatever exercise you do take should be vigorous enough to make you out of breath, otherwise it isn't doing you any good at all.

5 Try to avoid unnecessary stress. Take proper holidays – don't take work home with you – learn to relax.

6 If you are a woman, and over 40, don't use the pill if you have other 'risk factors' working against you. If you are a smoker, suffer from diabetes or have relatives with coronary artery disease, you would be wiser to use some other contraceptive method.

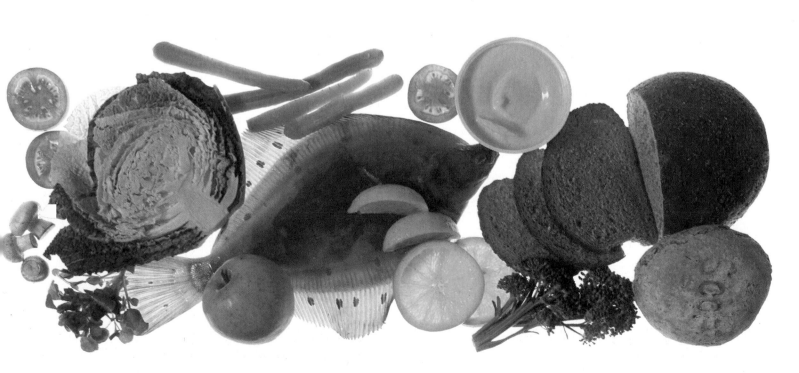

Below: A healthy diet is high in fruit and fibre foods; as low as possible in fat, meat and sugar.

CARING FOR
THE ELDERLY

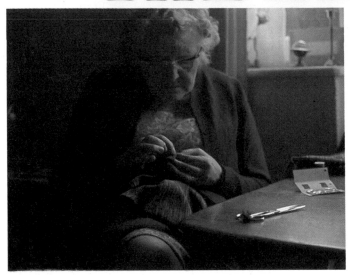

Above: Old people are especially accident-prone and may need help to make their homes as safe as possible.

After the age of 55 the accident rate rises quite steeply, and the older you are, the more vulnerable you become.

Old people are at risk because they become increasingly absent-minded. As their senses – sight, smell and hearing – fail they are less likely to be able to spot dangers, and because their reactions and their powers of co-ordination and balance are slow and inefficient, they are less likely to be able to avoid them. The old person may not notice the pair of shoes left lying on the stairs, or the step down from the front door in an unfamiliar house. And having tripped, he will be unable to save himself, and will fall. Old people (especially women) have brittle bones, and so any fall they do have is likely to be more serious than in someone younger and tougher. Falls in fact account for by far the most fatal accidents in old people.

Old people feel the cold because their bodies are less efficient at making heat. If they are living alone, or are short of money, they may just not be able to keep themselves warm enough during a cold winter spell. If they become extremely chilled they will gradually slip into a state of stupor or unconsciousness. Such chilling or 'hypothermia', will prove fatal if it is not discovered and dealt with in time.

In their efforts to keep warm, old people may boost their household heating with dangerous paraffin heaters, or warm their clothes too close to an open or unguarded fire. Because their eyesight is poor and their hands stiff and often shaky, they are much more accident-prone when doing simple everyday jobs around the house.

For them, the ideal solution is to live with their families, but this is not always possible or practicable, and in any case, many, if not most, old people like to hold on to their independence as long as possible. But there are plenty of safety-measures that you can take to make sure that if your elderly relatives or friends are living alone they avoid some of the obvious dangers. The best precaution of all is to see that they are visited regularly, are on the telephone if possible, or at least have some way of contacting friends or neighbours – perhaps even by putting a card in a window – in an emergency.

FALLS

Make sure that there are no worn patches in carpets or linoleum, and that all treads on the stair-carpet are firmly fixed. Take up any loose rugs, and if possible see that there are no trailing electric flexes around the room. If an old person has any pain or bruising, especially in a hip, after a fall, make sure they have an x-ray, even if the fall seemed fairly trivial. Handrails fitted to the bath, and on the wall beside the lavatory, make it much easier, and therefore safer, for an elderly person to pull himself up. It is a good idea, too, to put a non-slip mat *in* the bath (as well as making sure that the bathroom floor is not slippery, particularly when wet).

After any minor fall or accident, keep an eye on cuts or minor wounds. They will not heal quite as quickly as in a younger person, and are rather more liable to become infected.

BURNS AND SCALDS

Any old person who can afford it should have proper central heating in their home. If this isn't possible, make sure that any open fires – coal, gas or electric – are well guarded. At bed-time, suggest that night-clothes are warmed in an airing cupboard rather than in front of a fire – and make sure, in any case, that they are made of non-inflammable material.

ACCIDENTAL POISONING

Suggest that any pills or sleeping tablets are kept in a medicine chest rather than on the table by the bed. In a confused or sleepy state at night it is very easy to forget that the normal dose has already been taken, and to repeat it. Make sure that all pills are kept in their own, clearly marked container.

TALKING TO YOUR DOCTOR

A doctor is rather like a computer, in that the more relevant information you are able to feed into him, the better the answer you are likely to receive. Many people behave as though their doctor has second sight, so that when he asks what's wrong they think, even if they do not say, 'That's for *you* to find out.' It will speed things up for both of you if you have some idea of what it is your doctor will want to know.

1 Explain your problem as clearly and accurately as you can. Don't try to be brave and gloss over your symptoms. Pain is one of the most important symptoms and a key pointer in helping your doctor assess exactly what is wrong with you. He will want to know when the pain began, whether it is continuous or comes and goes, the degree of pain, the area of your body it covers. Give him as much information as you can and explain what it is that is *really* worrying you. Many of us go to our doctors with some trivial complaint when what we really want is advice about something else, possibly something which is causing us considerable anxiety but which for some reason or another we do not find it easy to mention. Your doctor may, for example, have satisfied himself that all you are suffering from is indigestion, but what he won't realize, unless you tell him, is that you have been worrying for weeks in case you have cancer, and as a result, he will probably fail to give you the reassurance you need.

2 *Ask* if you don't understand what the doctor tells you and, if it is still not clear, do not hesitate to *ask again* until you do understand.

3 If you are prescribed any medicines or tablets make sure you know exactly how often and for how long you are to take them. Tell your doctor immediately if they cause any unpleasant side effects.

4 It is always nicer for the doctor to examine a clean patient who is wearing clean socks/tights and under-clothes. If he asks you to take deep breaths while he is examining your chest with his stethoscope, turn your head away so as not to breathe all over him.

PREPARING FOR A HOME VISIT

If your doctor visits you or a member of your family at home see that the patient is wearing clean pyjamas/nightdress and that the bed and bedroom are tidied beforehand. Besides assisting the doctor it also helps make the patient feel better. Doctors like to examine patients from their right side, so if it isn't possible for both sides of the bed to be easily reached, try to make sure that he can stand on the right.

The doctor will also need the following:
● Soap and water to wash his hands and a clean towel.
● A flat surface covered with a clean towel so that he can lay out any instruments or sterile dressings.
● If any dressings are to be changed, have ready a polythene bag for the dirty dressings, and a covered bowl or kettle containing cooled, boiled water.

Below: Doctors on the whole are friendly — even the smallest patient need not be frightened of being examined.

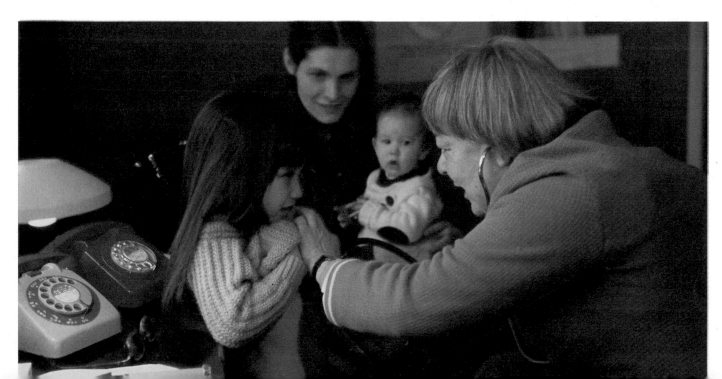

FIRST AID

WHAT TO KEEP IN YOUR FIRST AID BOX AND MEDICINE CHEST

Most people keep too much in their first aid kits, and far too much in their medicine cupboards. Your first aid kit should fit easily into a 4 litre (7 pint) polythene ice-cream carton. Your medicine chest would do the same, if it was confined to the things you actually *need*, but most of us tend to have a strong belief in the power of some patent medicine or other, and a magpie tendency to keep odds and ends of prescribed medicines, on the grounds that they are bound to come in useful when someone else in the family develops similar symptoms. Doctors usually prescribe a full course of medicine, which is meant to be finished. If you don't finish it, throw it away – medicine should be emptied down the sink, pills flushed down the loo since many drugs lose their effectiveness if they are kept too long. In any case you should NEVER give a medicine prescribed for one person to anyone else.

Your first aid box should contain:

1 box of adhesive plasters of assorted sizes, for minor cuts and grazes.

1 roll of porous synthetic surgical tape, for sticking on dressings, and for drawing together the edges of large cuts. This is much better than the standard zinc oxide plaster, to which many people are allergic.

2 large prepared wound dressings. 2 medium prepared wound dressings. Each packet contains dressings, pad and bandage. These are quick and easy to put on in an emergency.

1 packet non-adherent dry absorbent sterilized wound dressings. These are made with gauze instead of lint, and peel more easily off a wound.

1 packet sterilized cotton wool. This can be used to make swabs to clean wounds, or to provide padding around a wound.

2 or 3 tubular gauze bandages. These are much the easiest way to bandage fingers or toes.

2 large triangular bandages. These are used to make slings or, folded, to bind a dressing on to a wound.

1 standard crêpe bandage.

Safety pins, tweezers and scissors.

Your medicine chest should contain:

Soluble aspirin. Ask for 'soluble aspirin, B.P.' rather than a brand name; it's the same, and cheaper. Keep junior aspirin, if you have children. Aspirin is a pain-killing drug and will also help to bring a temperature down. Paracetamol, another popular pain-killing drug, is slightly more 'risky' than aspirin, since fewer tablets constitute an overdose. An overdose of paracetamol, even if it does not kill, can cause permanent liver damage.

● Anti-histamine cream. This is used for insect bites and stings.
● Calamine lotion. This can be used for sunburn and as an alternative to an anti-histamine cream for soothing insect bites or nettle stings.
● Travel sickness remedy. If you have travel-sick children, look for one that contains no hyoscine (the constituents will be printed on the packet).
● An antacid, to relieve indigestion.
● A bottle of kaolin and morphine, or kaolin and codeine mixture, for treating diarrhoea. For children, kaolin mixture alone is safest. This should be renewed every six months.
● A thermometer.
● A bottle of antiseptic solution for cleaning around wounds. Hydrogen peroxide can be used straight from the bottle. Most other antiseptic solutions must be diluted according to the directions on the bottle. If they are not carefully made up to the right strength they may damage the tissues, doing more harm than good. If no antiseptic is available, plain water, or soap and water, should be used.

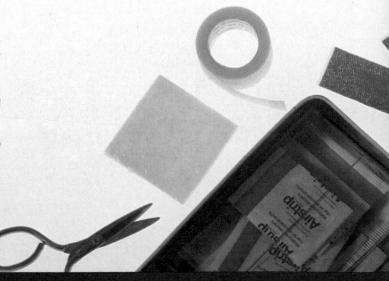

You can buy a first aid kit, but it is cheaper, and just as easy, to make up your own. The assortment of dressings and bandages shown here, together with one or two basic medicines such as aspirin, will enable you to deal with any minor accidents you or your family have.

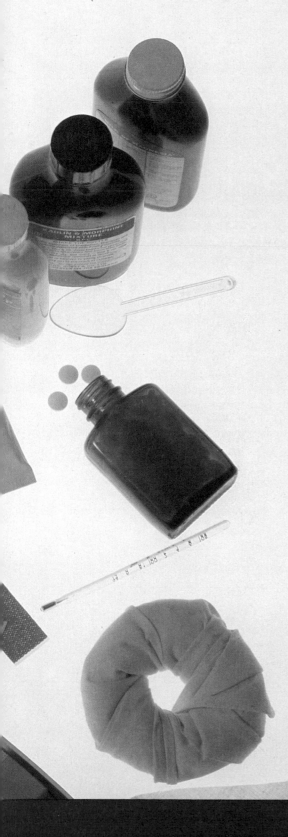

BASIC BANDAGING

Triangular bandages are probably one of the most useful since they can be used in so many different ways. The basic bandage is simply made by cutting a metre (39 in) square of calico across its diagonal. In an emergency you may have to improvise, and any plain material or even a scarf can be used.

To use a triangular bandage as a sling – for injuries to the ribs or arm:

1 Place bandage over front of body, taking one end behind the neck, forwards over the shoulder on the injured side. Support the weight of the injured arm carefully while you are doing this.

2 Place the injured arm over the bandage with the hand slightly higher than the elbow.

3 Bring the lower end of the bandage up, and tie both ends in a reef knot (left over right, then right over left). Turn the corner at the elbow forward, and pin or tuck it in. Leave the fingers exposed.

To improvise a sling:

If you do not have a scarf available, but need to support an injured arm, you can improvise by using a belt, tie or similar strap of material as a sling. If necessary you could also pin the sleeve of the sweater or coat being worn by the casualty to the front of the sweater or to the lapel of the coat.

To use a triangular bandage as a broad-fold bandage – to cover a large area, hold dressings in place or to immobilize a fracture – open up the bandage and fold the point over to meet the base. Then fold the bandage in half again. To use a triangular bandage as a narrow-fold bandage – to hold a pad in place over an eye – fold in half yet again.

To make a ring bandage, make one end of a narrow-fold bandage into a loop. Pass the other end through the loop and then wrap it round and round the loop until the whole of the bandage is used and a firm ring is made.

When bandaging any injury, always support the injured part so that the patient is comfortable. Bandage from below the injury upwards – start by pointing the end of the bandage obliquely upwards; a firm turn around this fixes the bandage securely. When applying a bandage, try to do it firmly and evenly, with each turn covering two-thirds of the previous one.

ANIMAL BITES & STINGS

Although an animal bite may not look, or even feel, particularly serious, it is a potential source of infection. The teeth of cats and dogs may harbour particularly dangerous germs, such as those that cause tetanus for example, and because the wound is made with sharp pointed teeth, these germs can penetrate quite deeply into the body. So, however innocuous a bite may appear, there is a considerable risk, not only that the wound itself may become locally infected, but that a more general infection may be spread throughout the body. It is for this reason that you should only treat very minor, surface bites and scratches yourself – deeper, more serious bites should be shown to a doctor. Outside the UK, in countries where rabies may be present, ANY bite from a warm-blooded animal, whether domestic or wild, should be shown to a doctor straight away.

ANIMAL BITES

1 Superficial bites and scratches by dogs and cats, that have only just broken the skin, are safe to treat at home. Simply wash around the wound with soap and water, or hydrogen peroxide, pat dry and cover with a sterile, dry dressing. Keep an eye on the wound over the next day or two in case it becomes infected. If the surrounding skin starts to look red or seems tender or there are any signs of pus, or if you are in any doubt whatsoever, consult a doctor. This is particularly important for bites on the face and bites by cats.

2 Don't try to treat a serious bite yourself, especially a deep puncture wound caused by a dog's teeth.

Wash the area with soap and water or hydrogen peroxide and get to a doctor or hospital casualty department as soon as you can. Such wounds are likely to become infected if not properly treated. Your doctor may give you a course of antibiotic treatment and possibly an anti-tetanus injection.

3 If you are in a country where rabies may be present (which means most countries outside the UK), *any* animal bite, whether it is from a wild animal or a domestic dog or cat, should be washed immediately and then shown to a doctor. You may need to be given a course of anti-rabies injections – if this is done promptly it can effectively prevent the disease.

SNAKE BITES

The adder is the only poisonous British snake. It will never attack but it may bite if you step on it. Its bite is seldom serious, though it may be dangerous for the very old or the very young. Adder bites hurt, and because many people are terrified by snakes, they may be dangerously SHOCKED by being bitten (p. 69) even though there is little or no poison in the wound.

1 Calm and reassure the patient and make him either sit or lie down – walking around will help spread the poison, if there is any, around the body.

Below: An adder can grow up to 711 mm (28 in) long and has a thick body with a V-shaped mark at the back of its head and a diamond pattern along its back. It is found on dry moors and sunny hillsides.

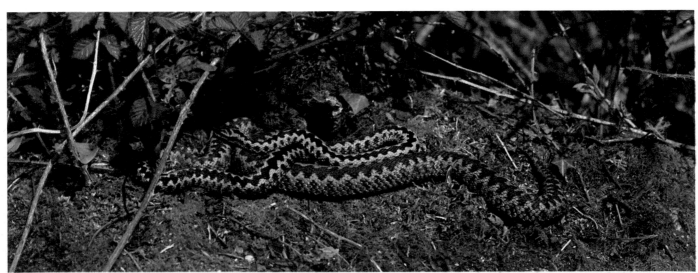

2 Wash the wound with soapy water and put a dry, sterile dressing over it.

3 Keep the part of the body that has been bitten as still as possible.

4 Watch for signs of SHOCK (p. 69). If the patient seems pale, faint, sweaty, dizzy or very shaken lie him down with his feet raised and keep him warm (though not too warm).

5 Get the patient to a doctor or hospital casualty department as soon as possible.

STINGS

For most people, insect and plant stings cause nothing more serious than some local swelling, pain or itchiness, and redness of the skin around the sting. Bee and wasp stings and horsefly bites usually produce the worst reactions. A few people may show a more serious *allergic reaction*, which can affect the whole of their body. This may provoke an attack of DIFFICULT BREATHING (p. 52), or asthma; produce a general skin rash with large, weal-like swellings; or a shock-like reaction, with faintness, pallor and sweating. Once you have experienced this sort of generalized reaction to a sting, even though it was fairly mild, you are likely to react in the same way, but more seriously, the next time you are stung. Anyone who shows an allergic reaction to a sting should see a doctor immediately – a serious reaction can be life-threatening. Otherwise you can treat the sting yourself.

INSECT STINGS

1 If you are stung by a bee the sting, with the poison sac, will possibly have been left in the skin. If you, or a companion, can see the sting, pull it out with a pair of eyebrow tweezers. Do not express by squeezing as this spreads the poison.

2 There is no basis for the old 'acid for a wasp sting, alkali for a bee' theory. An anti-histamine cream, if you apply it immediately, is the most effective way to reduce itching, otherwise any form of cooling will help to soothe the pain. Surgical spirit, because it evaporates quickly from the skin, works well but calamine lotion or ice-packs may prove just as effective.

3 Bee or wasp stings inside the mouth can be especially nasty and can cause severe swelling which may interfere with breathing. Give the patient sips of the coldest drink possible; if available, ice cubes are ideal to suck. Get him to a doctor straight away.

NETTLE STINGS

There is no proven medical reason for treating nettle stings with dock leaves except that they are cool and therefore soothing. But children, especially, like to be treated immediately with something and, on a country walk, dock leaves are likely to be the most immediately

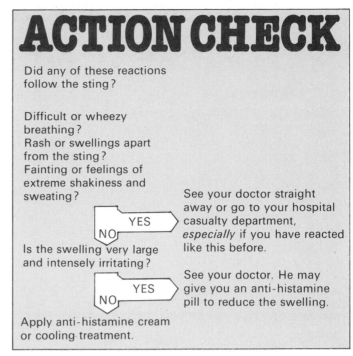

ACTION CHECK

Did any of these reactions follow the sting?

Difficult or wheezy breathing?
Rash or swellings apart from the sting?
Fainting or feelings of extreme shakiness and sweating?

YES / NO

See your doctor straight away or go to your hospital casualty department, *especially* if you have reacted like this before.

Is the swelling very large and intensely irritating?

YES / NO

See your doctor. He may give you an anti-histamine pill to reduce the swelling.

Apply anti-histamine cream or cooling treatment.

available treatment. By the time you reach home the irritation will probably have subsided; if not, calamine lotion, anti-histamine cream or an ice-pack will soothe the stings and reduce the inflammation.

JELLYFISH STINGS

Stings from jellyfish found around the British coast cause painful burning and swelling but are seldom serious. Treat them with anti-histamine cream, calamine lotion or ice-packs. The only dangerous jellyfish in European waters is the pale blue Portuguese man-of-war, whose stinging tentacles stick to the skin. If you are stung by one of these, you should scrape off the tentacles using wet sand and seek medical help as quickly as possible.

Below: The Portuguese man-of-war, often referred to as a 'jellyfish', is in fact a colony of animals. Renowned for its powerful sting, it was formerly known as a sea nettle.

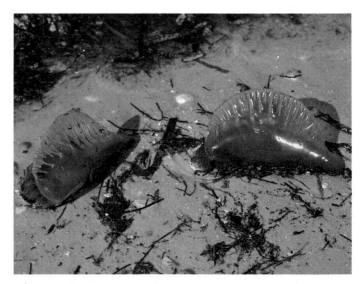

BLEEDING

Blood cannot clot while it is flowing freely, and while an adult can lose over a pint of blood without any ill effects, heavier blood loss can result in SHOCK (p. 69) and can be life-threatening. For infants and children, whose total blood volume is much less, a loss of even half a pint is dangerous.

1 Make the casualty lie down and raise the injured part if you can – this will reduce the blood flow through it.

2 Press hard on the wound, using a pad made of a clean folded handkerchief or a folded bandage or dressing. If nothing else is available, press with your fingers, drawing the edges of the wound firmly together if you can. Maintain the pressure for about ten minutes, by which time a clot should have begun to form.

3 As soon as the blood flow stops, pick out any *loose* dirt or foreign bodies in the wound but don't attempt to probe for anything that is deeply embedded.

4 Apply a clean pad or dressing, binding it firmly on with a bandage. If there is any obvious foreign body embedded or protruding from the wound, don't put the dressing directly over it but apply a ring bandage (p. 33), or put padding around the area so that there is no direct pressure on it.

5 If blood oozes through the dressing, don't remove it but put another one on top.

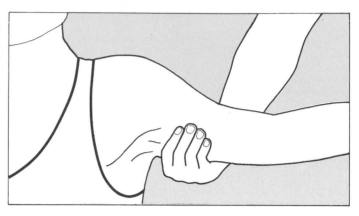

Above: Stop severe bleeding in the arm by pressing hard against the inner side of the upper arm. This is roughly along the line of the inner seam of a coat sleeve.

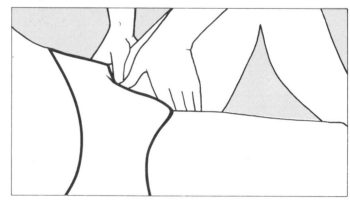

Above: Firm pressure with both thumbs at the mid-point of the groin will compress the femoral artery against the bone and stop severe bleeding in the leg.

PRESSURE POINTS

If simple direct pressure fails to stop the bleeding and the wound is in an arm or a leg you may be able to stop it by pressing the bleeding artery against a bone. If the bleeding is in the hand or lower arm, press the inner side of the upper arm hard against the bone. If it is in the lower leg, bend the casualty's knee and press with both thumbs, one on top of the other, at the centre of the fold of the groin. This 'indirect pressure' should not be applied for longer than 15 minutes.

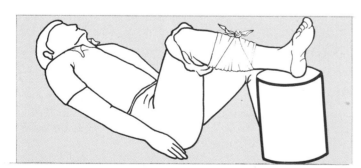

Above: Raising an injured limb will help to stop bleeding by slowing down the blood flow.

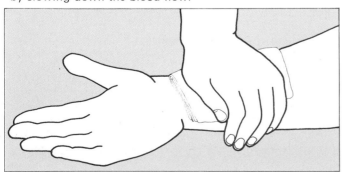

NEVER
Never make a tourniquet by tying anything around the limb. This is a very risky procedure which could lead to the loss of the limb.

Left: The flow of blood from a wound can usually be staunched by direct pressure, using a folded pad or bandage.

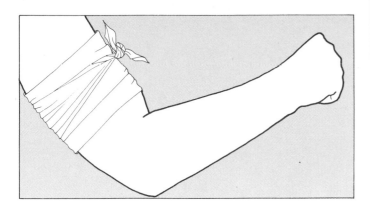

Above: Once bleeding has stopped, bandage a clean pad over the wound, using a scarf or triangular bandage. Tie knot on uninjured side.

Below: Wounds in the palm of the hand bleed freely. Hold a pad over the cut with fingers clenched, then bandage around the whole hand.

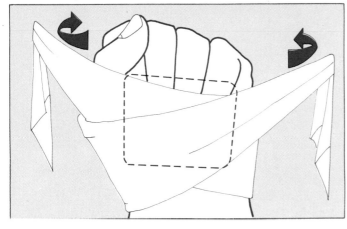

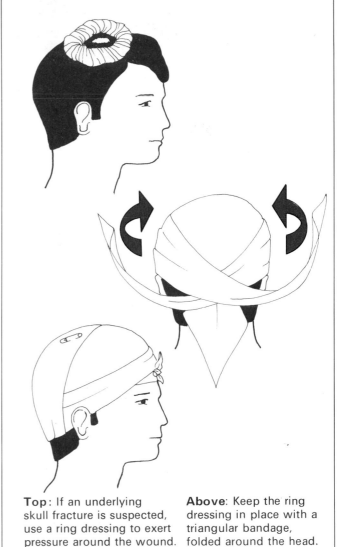

Top: If an underlying skull fracture is suspected, use a ring dressing to exert pressure around the wound.

Above: Keep the ring dressing in place with a triangular bandage, folded around the head.

SCALP WOUNDS

These often bleed very heavily but you should not apply direct pressure in case there is an underlying fracture of the skull. If you feel sure there is no fracture, bandage a large dressing firmly on. If you suspect there may be a fracture, put on a ring dressing so there is pressure around the area, but not directly on the wound. (See p. 33).

GUNSHOT WOUNDS

Although the entry wound made by a bullet may be quite small, the exit wound is likely to be large and bleed heavily and the passage of the bullet may also cause extensive internal injuries. Bandage or pack with a large dressing. It is vital for a doctor to see such a wound as soon as possible.

BLISTERS

A blister is formed when the outermost layer of skin becomes separated from the inner layers by a fluid-filled 'bubble'. As the skin beneath heals, the fluid is re-absorbed and the surface layer of dead skin peels away. Blisters are caused either by rubbing or by BURNS (p. 43). New or badly-fitting shoes, or shoes worn without socks, are the most usual causes of friction-blisters.

1 Leave the blister alone. Its function is to protect the new skin below. So don't prick, squeeze or tear off the top skin.

2 If the blister is going to be exposed to further rubbing, for example if it is on a foot, protect it with an adhesive dressing.

BROKEN BONES & DISLOCATIONS

Although a dislocation is an injury to a joint rather than a bone, it is easier to discuss breaks and dislocations together because it is not always possible to decide with which you are dealing. Both may have very similar symptoms and the general first aid treatment is the same in either case.

A bone can break (fracture) either as the result of a direct blow, or by indirect 'jarring'. For example, the collar-bone, which is a fairly slender bone, is easily fractured by a fall on to an outstretched hand.

The different types of fracture are:

1 An OPEN fracture is one in which the broken bone has penetrated the skin, so that there is an open wound. This is the most serious type because of the danger of infection.

2 In a CLOSED fracture there is no open wound. If the fracture has caused internal bleeding or damage to internal organs it is called a complicated fracture.

3 Because the bones of children are more soft and pliable than those of adults, they may bend rather than break, producing the partial break called a GREENSTICK fracture.

As people get older their bones become increasingly fragile; even a minor fall may fracture a bone in an elderly person.

Sometimes, it is quite obvious after an accident that a limb is broken because it is misshapen. Often, it is impossible to tell without an x-ray whether there is a fracture or whether the limb is just badly bruised or a joint sprained. If there are no obvious signs of a fracture you can treat the injury simply by resting it for a few hours to see if the pain and bruising subside.

A DISLOCATION is the wrenching out of place of one or more bones at a joint. The shoulder joint is the one most easily displaced but knees, elbows, fingers, thumb and lower jaw are also easily dislocated.

The symptoms of breaks and dislocations are:

Severe pain, swelling, inability to move the injured part without great pain, or to control it normally; deformity – especially noticeable if a bone is dislocated. A broken limb may be lying at an odd angle or look slightly shorter than the uninjured one. SHOCK (p. 69) very often follows a serious fracture or dislocation.

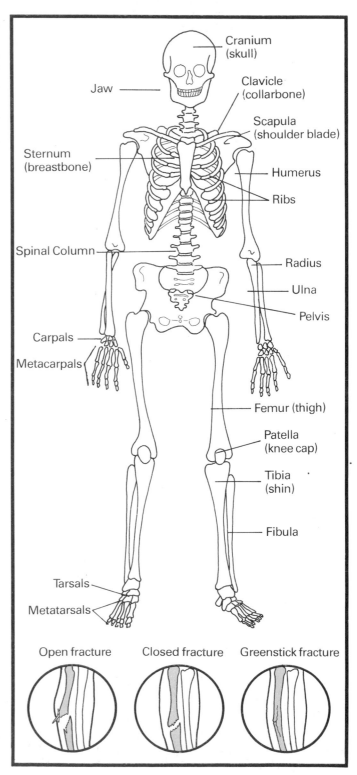

Cranium (skull)

Jaw

Clavicle (collarbone)

Scapula (shoulder blade)

Sternum (breastbone)

Humerus

Ribs

Spinal Column

Radius

Ulna

Pelvis

Carpals

Metacarpals

Femur (thigh)

Patella (knee cap)

Tibia (shin)

Fibula

Tarsals

Metatarsals

Open fracture   Closed fracture   Greenstick fracture

Broken bones need medical attention. By moving the bones – or the patient – you may do even more damage and almost certainly cause a lot more pain.

So, do *not* try to move the patient. Your aim should be to get help as quickly as you can and to make the patient as comfortable as you can while you are waiting for it. If he complains of pain in his back or neck, or has any loss of power or feeling in his hands or feet, it is doubly important for you not to move him. He may have fractured his spine and you run the risk of damaging the spinal cord and causing a permanent paralysis if you bend or twist his back or neck.

However, there may be times when help is not instantly available, particularly after an accident on a walking or mountaineering trip. In these circumstances you may need to take more positive action, by immobilizing and padding the broken part so that the patient can be transported as comfortably as possible.

IF HELP IS NOT IMMEDIATELY AVAILABLE

1 DON'T move the patient (unless he is in any real danger where he is), but treat him on the spot.

2 Cover any open wound.

3 If there is severe bleeding because the ends of a broken bone have pierced the skin, you will not be able to control it in the usual way by applying direct pressure. Instead, you must apply pressure ALONGSIDE the broken bone, or press the edges of the wound gently but firmly together.

4 DON'T try to move the casualty until you have immobilized the injured part. Move the limb into the most comfortable position you can (see *Immobilizing Broken Limbs* p. 40) and then bandage it to the casualty's body to support it and keep it still. Use belts, scarves, ties – whatever is available – to do this, and fasten the limb so that the joints above and below the break are both immobilized. Rolled-up newspapers or magazines can be used as improvised splints to give extra rigidity.

5 Use lots of padding around the limb and between any areas of skin. Here again, use whatever is available – folded sweaters, anoraks or any spare clothing. A rolled blanket or towel, or a pillow folded and tied around the limb, will act as both splint and padding.

6 Raise the injured part – this will help to reduce pain and swelling.

7 Try to prevent SHOCK (p. 69). Loosen any tight clothing around the casualty's neck and waist, and cover him with a coat or blanket to prevent chilling.

8 DON'T GIVE ANYTHING to eat or drink – if a bone has to be set, a general anaesthetic will be needed.

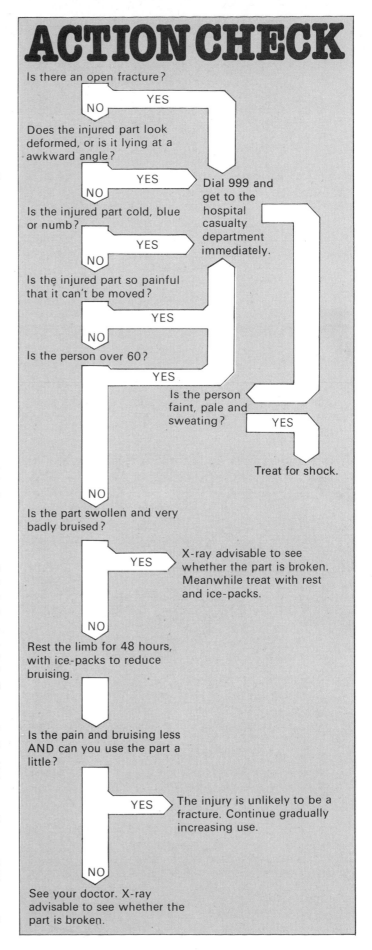

ACTION CHECK

Is there an open fracture?

NO — YES

Does the injured part look deformed, or is it lying at a awkward angle?

NO — YES

Is the injured part cold, blue or numb?

NO — YES

Dial 999 and get to the hospital casualty department immediately.

Is the injured part so painful that it can't be moved?

NO — YES

Is the person over 60?

NO — YES

Is the person faint, pale and sweating?

YES

Treat for shock.

Is the part swollen and very badly bruised?

NO — YES

X-ray advisable to see whether the part is broken. Meanwhile treat with rest and ice-packs.

Rest the limb for 48 hours, with ice-packs to reduce bruising.

Is the pain and bruising less AND can you use the part a little?

NO — YES

The injury is unlikely to be a fracture. Continue gradually increasing use.

See your doctor. X-ray advisable to see whether the part is broken.

IMMOBILIZING BROKEN LIMBS
Broken arm or collar bone

The person will usually automatically support the arm in whatever position is most comfortable, cradling it across his chest in the uninjured arm.

1 Support the weight of the arm in a sling (for improvised slings see p. 33). Put plenty of soft padding between the arm and the body. Use whatever soft clothing or material you can find. For extra rigidity, particularly when there is a long journey involved, pass a belt or tie over the sling and around the body to fix the arm in position.

2 If an elbow is broken the arm may be held bent or straight. If bent, support the arm in a sling as above. If straight, immobilize it by tying to the side of the casualty's body with belts, ties or scarves.

3 If a hand is injured, protect it in a fold of soft padding and then put the arm in a sling.

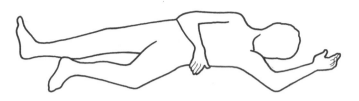

Above: If a thigh is fractured, the casualty's injured leg and foot will be turned outwards.

Below: Fasten padded splints in place with ties around legs and body, positioning the last bandage just below the break.

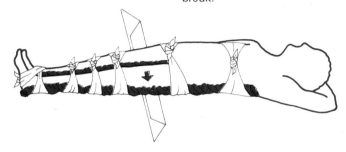

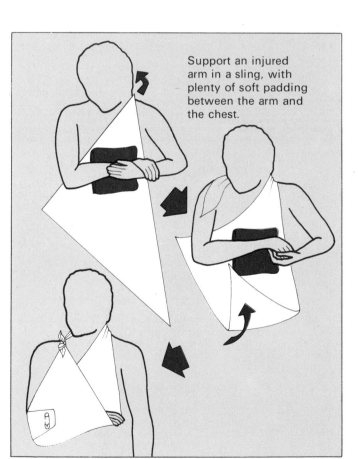

Support an injured arm in a sling, with plenty of soft padding between the arm and the chest.

DON'T

Don't tie the bandages too tightly, just firmly enough to keep the limb still. Bandages must never be put over the site of the fracture but above and below it.

Broken leg or thigh

If the accident happens in a home environment, do not move the casualty unnecessarily, but make him as comfortable as possible until medical help arrives.

1 Straighten the legs slowly and gently so as to bring them in line with each other as much as possible without causing the patient too much pain.

2 Put plenty of padding between the thighs, knees and ankles. A folded blanket or rolled-up towels wrapped around the limb and between the legs will act as a combined splint and padding.

3 Bind the injured limb to the undamaged one, with whatever belts, scarves or ties are available. Make one tie at the knee and the other as a figure of eight around feet and ankles.

4 If you have a long or difficult journey to hospital, the casualty will be more comfortable if you use extra bandages to bind the limb at thigh, leg and just below the site of the break, and if you can improvise some sort of splint to give extra rigidity. If a piece of board is not available, use rolled-up newspapers or, even better, magazines. Put these, again with plenty of padding, between his legs.

5 If a *thigh* is injured, try to find something to make an additional padded splint on the outer side of the limb, from ankle to armpit, secured with two additional bandages around the chest and hips.

6 Check the bandages every quarter of an hour – swelling of the limb may cause them to become too tight. Always tie knots on the uninjured side of the body, and always use reef knots (left over right, then right over left).

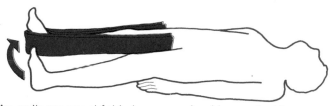

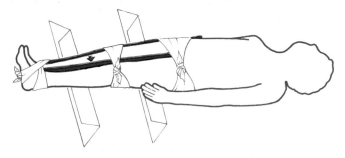

An ordinary towel folded around a broken leg will act as both splint and padding. Tie injured leg to the good one at feet and ankles, and add extra ties at thigh, leg and just below the break if there is a difficult journey ahead.

Fractured spine

If you suspect that someone may have a fractured spine DO NOT MOVE HIM. If he is conscious, the person may complain of severe pain in his back or neck, together with some loss of feeling or control over his limbs. Moving someone with this kind of injury is a difficult and specialized job, calling for at least four experienced, qualified first-aiders and a rigid stretcher. It is unlikely that you will have this sort of assistance available, so until such help arrives, leave the casualty where he is, cover him with a coat or blanket to keep him warm, and above all, KEEP HIM STILL.

If, in a real emergency, the danger of moving him is less risky than leaving him where he is (perhaps because the roof of a building is in imminent danger of caving in), you should try to *drag* him away from danger on his back on a coat or blanket so that you keep him as flat as possible. If possible have a helper to pull on his feet to keep his spine straight. YOU SHOULD ONLY ATTEMPT THIS IN A *REAL* EMERGENCY, WHERE A LIFE IS AT STAKE.

Fractured jaw

1 Remove any loose or false teeth.

2 Support the jaw with a pad beneath the chin held in place either by hand or with a bandage tied on top of the head.

3 Help the person to sit with his head well forward. If he should want to vomit, slip off the bandage but support his chin with your hand.

4 If the casualty is severely injured or unconscious, place in the RECOVERY POSITION (p. 73).

The knee

Any knee injury serious enough to cause severe pain or to limit the movement of the joint should be seen by a doctor or the patient taken to a casualty department. If a cartilage within the knee has been torn or displaced by a sudden blow or wrench the knee may be held fixed in a bent position – any attempt to straighten it will cause severe pain. A blow on the knee may fracture the kneecap. The joint will be very painful and you may be able to feel the two halves of the kneecap.

1 Lay the casualty on his back with his head and shoulders raised.

2 Raise and support the injured leg.

3 Put a splint, using rolled-up newspapers or magazines if no piece of board is available, along the back of the leg, extending from the top of the thigh to just beyond the heel. Put plenty of padding around the splint, especially in the hollows of the knee and ankle.

4 Bind the leg to the splint with bandages around the thigh, below the knee and around the ankle and foot.

5 Keep the injured leg propped up.

DISLOCATION
Fingers

A finger may sometimes become dislocated, usually at the base of the knuckle nearest to the palm. You may be able to reposition this yourself. Pull the finger to straighten it and then push gently sideways until it clicks into position. DON'T force it – if it doesn't click back easily, see a doctor.

Shoulder

A shoulder joint is easily dislocated because the socket into which the bone of the arm (this is called the humerus) fits, is very shallow. When a shoulder is dislocated, the arm is usually forced forwards and inwards. Do not try to push the joint back into place, but support the arm in a sling and seek medical help.

Below: Because the normal shoulder joint (left) is very shallow, the head of the humerus may become dislocated, slipping downwards and forwards as shown (right).

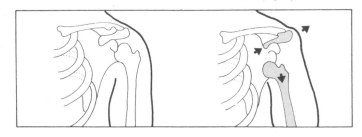

BRUISES

A bruise is the result of bleeding into the tissues beneath the skin, after a fall or a blow. The bruise looks swollen and blue-black at first, then the swelling gradually subsides and the discoloration fades to a greenish-yellow before finally disappearing. A bruise in a place where the underlying bone is near the skin surface – on the shin, for example, or the head – may swell dramatically but this doesn't mean that it is any more serious than a normal bruise; it just looks worse. Trivial bruising needs no treatment, but the pain and swelling on a badly bruised area can be reduced by applying a cold compress or an ice-pack.

COLD COMPRESS TREATMENT

Soak a handkerchief, wad of cotton wool, or piece of flannel or towelling – in fact any reasonably absorbent material – in cold (preferably iced) water. Place it over the bruise, holding it in place with a length of open weave bandage, but don't cover it, so that the water can evaporate freely. Keep the compress on the bruise for about half an hour – if it dries out, dampen it again. You can make an ice-pack by filling a polythene bag two-thirds full of a mixture of crushed ice and salt. Squeeze the air out, tie the bag and wrap it in a thin towel or tea-cloth. Picnic freezer-bags, which retain their coldness after an initial cooling period in the ice-compartment or freezer, also make good ice-packs.

BLACK EYES

A blow to the skin around the eye can produce spectacular bruising and swelling in the eyelids and surrounding tissue. The eye itself is seldom damaged by such a blow, because it is protected by being set well back in a bony socket, but it is advisable to check with a doctor that all is well, and this is essential if you have any visual disturbance following the injury.

OLD WIVES' TALE

The traditional remedy for a black eye was to use a piece of steak as a cold compress. However, even the best quality fillet steak has no magical healing properties.

BURNS & SCALDS

The heat from a burn or scald not only damages the skin itself but also the blood vessels that lie below the skin's surface so that the colourless fluid, or plasma, which forms most of the volume of the blood, begins to leak. The larger the area of skin affected by the burn, the larger the volume of lost plasma will be. If a lot of plasma is lost, the volume of circulating blood may be considerably reduced producing a state of SHOCK (p. 69). A burn that covers 10% or more of the body area – that is, an area the size of the back, or the chest, or one whole arm – is likely to cause shock because of loss of plasma. The severity of a burn is judged more by the area that it covers than by its depth. Large superficial burns, which only damage the outer layers of the skin, can in fact be more painful than small deep burns which destroy the whole thickness of the skin, because the nerve endings that are sensitive to pain are situated in the outer layers of the skin.

Besides shock, the main danger from burns is infection. Any burn that affects more than a few square centimetres of skin should be seen by a doctor. In children or babies all but the smallest burns should be seen by a doctor. If the burned area is large or the burns are deep, you should summon an ambulance and get the casualty to hospital immediately.

First aid treatment for all burns and scalds is the same. Cool the whole area as quickly as possible, by drenching it with cold water and continue cooling it for at least 10 minutes, or until the pain stops. For minor 'cooking burns', which are usually small and superficial, this is all the treatment that should be necessary. Cooling relieves the pain and helps to stop plasma loss by closing up the damaged blood vessels. Remove anything constricting, for example rings, belts or shoes, before the area starts to swell.

1 If the skin is SCALDED with hot water or oil and if you are on the spot to give first aid treatment within minutes of the accident, remove any covering clothing quickly before you cool the area. Otherwise the clothing will act like a poultice and by keeping the heat in will do further damage. If by the time you arrive on the scene the clothing has cooled, don't remove it.

2 Don't remove clothing that has been BURNT. Burnt clothing will be sterile and will be some protection against infection.

3 DO remove any clothing that is soaked in corrosive chemicals, acid or alkali. PROTECT your own hands while you are doing this.

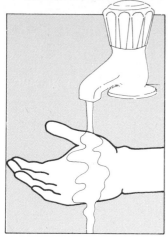

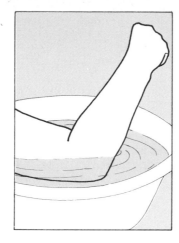

Above left: Holding a burn under cold running water will reduce pain and swelling.

Above right: For a burn covering a large area, immerse the whole limb in cold water.

4 If you are only dealing with a small burn, hold it under a running cold tap. Otherwise drench the area with cold water and maintain this with wet cloths. Change the cloths as they lose their coldness. Keep up the cooling treatment for at least ten minutes.

5 Gently remove any rings, belts, bracelets or anything constricting from the burnt area. Later, after the part has swollen, it will be more difficult to remove them.

6 If the burn covers more than about 20 cm^2 (3 sq. in), or if it is on the face or hands where scarring should be avoided, it needs medical treatment. Cover the area with a sterile dressing. In an emergency you can use the *inside* of a clean, ironed handkerchief, pillowcase or sheet. If fluid leaks through the dressing add another layer of dressing on top. The aim is to stop the plasma coming in contact with the air and forming a route for infection. Make sure that whatever you use for a dressing is non-fluffy. Do not use lint. A non-adherent dry absorbent dressing, held in place with a loose bandage, is the best.

7 The badly burned person may suffer from SHOCK (p. 69). Lie the patient down and keep him warm. You can give him small sips of water (burns are the only serious injury for which you can safely offer a drink), but don't give the traditional cup of hot, sweet tea.

8 When blisters form, don't prick them – they protect the underlying wound from infection. If a blister bursts, don't cut off the dead skin. It will still give some protection.

OLD WIVES' TALE

Never put oil, butter, flour or anything other than water on to a burn. It won't help and will have to be cleaned off the skin later, perhaps damaging the area even more.

ACTION CHECK

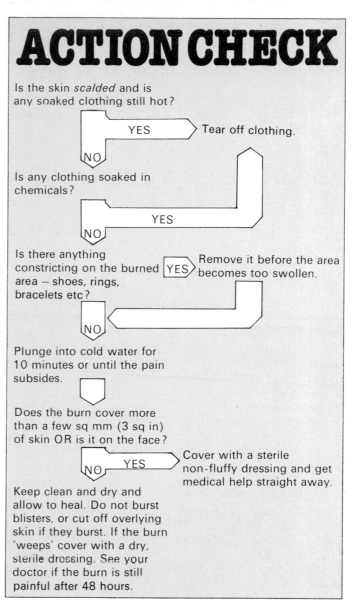

Is the skin *scalded* and is any soaked clothing still hot?

YES → Tear off clothing.

NO

Is any clothing soaked in chemicals?

YES

NO

Is there anything constricting on the burned area – shoes, rings, bracelets etc? YES → Remove it before the area becomes too swollen.

NO

Plunge into cold water for 10 minutes or until the pain subsides.

Does the burn cover more than a few sq mm (3 sq in) of skin OR is it on the face?

NO   YES → Cover with a sterile non-fluffy dressing and get medical help straight away.

Keep clean and dry and allow to heal. Do not burst blisters, or cut off overlying skin if they burst. If the burn 'weeps' cover with a dry, sterile dressing. See your doctor if the burn is still painful after 48 hours.

DON'T

Don't allow anyone whose clothing has caught fire to rush outside into the open. Air will fan the flames. Throw him to the floor (because fire rises) and smother the flames with a rug or blanket – away from the direction of his face if possible. Don't roll him round and round in a rug in your efforts to smother the flames. This will expose more of his body to the flames.

ELECTRICAL BURNS

Electrical burns may look smaller and more trivial than they really are, for the electrical current can penetrate deep into the skin tissues and seriously damage them. Any electrical burn should be seen by a doctor. First aid treatment is by cold water cooling. Someone who has had a bad electric shock may be suffering from shock, may be unconscious or have stopped breathing. If so, the treatment of any of these takes priority over first aid treatment for burns. (ELECTRIC SHOCK, p. 54).

CHILDBIRTH (EMERGENCY)

Only doctors and state-certified midwives are allowed by law to undertake maternity work. So only in exceptional circumstances, should you intervene.

Miscarriage

Although it is very unlikely that you will ever have to deliver a baby yourself, the chances of your having to render first aid to someone who is miscarrying are very much higher. About one pregnancy in every seven ends in a miscarriage, which is the termination of a pregnancy with delivery of the fetus before the 28th week. The proper medical term for miscarriage is 'spontaneous abortion'. About three-quarters of all such abortions are nature's way of getting rid of an embryo which is not developing properly: they are *not* caused by shock, excitement or by lifting heavy weights. Occasionally a miscarriage may follow a severe illness or be the result of an abnormality of the womb (uterus) or weakness of the mouth of the womb (cervix).

Most miscarriages occur in the first three months of pregnancy and are accompanied by bleeding from the vagina; this may be quite slight, or as heavy as a normal period. There is sometimes pain in the lower back or lower part of the abdomen. ANY bleeding or abdominal pain during pregnancy should be treated as follows:

1 Make the patient lie down immediately. She should not move until she has been seen by a doctor.

2 Send for the doctor.

Below: During labour the most effective and comfortable position is propped up against pillows, the knees drawn up and chin tucked in.

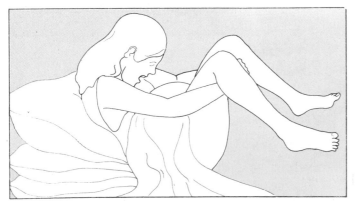

3 Give the patient a sanitary towel, but NO internal protection, e.g. Tampax, etc.

The most important point to remember if you ever have to deliver a baby without any medical help is to do as little as possible. Once the birth process has begun there is nothing you can do either to speed things up or to slow them down. The baby will be born come what may. A large part of your job will be to comfort and reassure the mother, who is likely to be at least as apprehensive at the lack of a doctor or midwife as you are yourself, especially if this is her first baby.

LABOUR

Labour can begin in one of three ways:

● The onset of regular 'labour pains' or contractions. These are usually felt in the lower part of the abdomen and sometimes across the lower part of the back.
● A discharge of blood-stained mucus called a 'show'.
● Occasionally by the 'breaking of the waters', i.e. the rupture of the bag of fluid that surrounds the baby. This can vary from a trickle to a gush of clear fluid.

Labour has three distinct stages. During the first stage the mouth of the womb (cervix) widens to permit the passage of the baby. This stage lasts for several hours. During the second stage the muscles of the uterus contract to push the baby through the birth canal. This stage, which culminates in the birth, seldom lasts longer than an hour for a first baby and can be very much shorter in subsequent births. The third stage is the expulsion of the afterbirth, or placenta, usually 10–15 minutes after the birth.

1 During the first stage, make the following preparations. Sterilize a pair of scissors and 4, 200 mm (9 in) lengths of string, either by boiling for 10 minutes or soaking in methylated spirits for 10 minutes. Protect the bed (or other flat surface if no bed is available) with a clean sheet over a layer of newspaper or a plastic sheet. Fold a blanket into three and wrap it in a clean sheet. This will cover the woman's top half during the delivery, while leaving her bottom half free. You will also need a soft towel or blanket to wrap the baby in, and a couple of covered basins of previously boiled water, with clean cloths or swabs, to clean up the mother and to wipe the baby's face. Make sure that your own hands are scrubbed clean.

ACTION CHECK

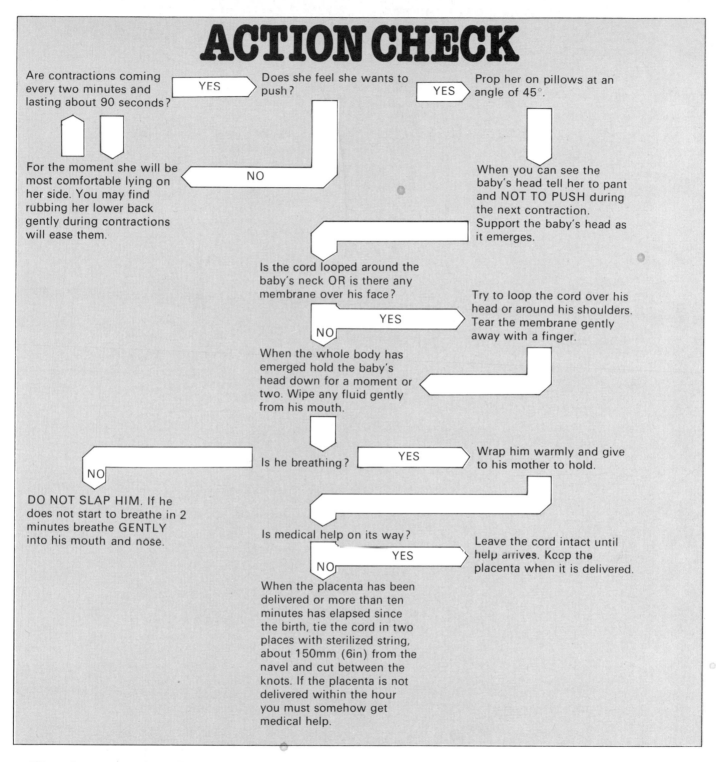

2 Time the contractions. By the end of the first stage they will be coming every two minutes and lasting about 90 seconds. During the first stage the woman will probably be most comfortable lying on her side.

3 At the beginning of the second stage the woman will feel an irresistible urge to push, as though pushing out a bowel movement. She will be most comfortable and be able to push most effectively if you prop her against pillows at an angle of about 45°. During each contraction tell her to draw her knees up and tuck her head down. If a bowel movement occurs, wipe it away from front to back, so that it cannot soil the birth canal.

4 Watch at each contraction until you see a bulge between her legs which is the crown of the baby's head stretching the vaginal entrance. When you see this, tell the woman NOT TO PUSH during the next contraction, but to take short, panting breaths with her mouth open. If she were to push vigorously now, the baby would be forced out too quickly and the mother's surrounding tissue (perineum) might be badly torn as a result. Tell her that she can, if she likes, push gently *between* contractions.

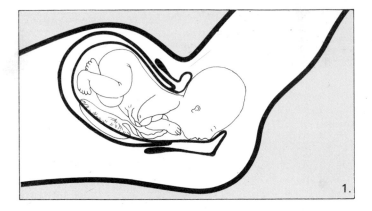

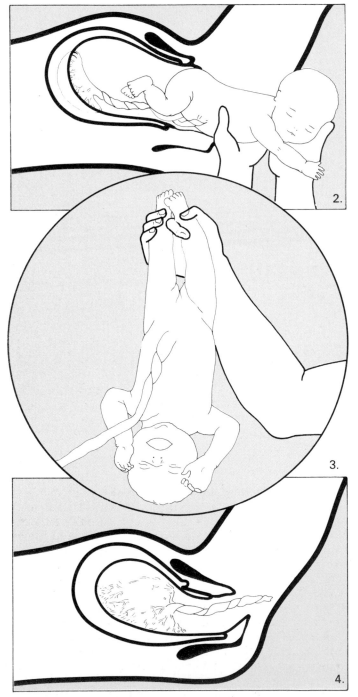

5 As the baby's head emerges, support it in your hands but do not pull. If you can see a membrane over the baby's face, tear it off gently with a finger. If the umbilical cord is around the baby's neck, try to hook it gently over his head or loop it over a shoulder.

6 Once the head is born, the shoulders and body will slide quickly out. Lift the baby, being careful NOT TO PULL ON THE CORD, wrap a cloth around his ankles (because he will be very slippery) and hold him head downwards for a moment or two, so that any fluid can drain from his mouth and nose. Wipe his mouth gently with a clean swab.

7 DO NOT slap him on the back. If he does not start to breathe of his own accord within two minutes, breathe *very gently* into his mouth and nose, watching his chest to see when he does begin to breathe.

8 Wrap the baby warmly before giving him to his mother to hold. A new-born baby easily becomes chilled.

9 The placenta should be delivered 10–15 minutes after the baby. Keep it – the doctor will want to examine the placenta to make sure that none has been left inside the uterus. There will be some bleeding after the placenta is expelled, but if the bleeding seems very heavy, massage the mother's abdomen, just below her navel. This will encourage the uterus to contract again, closing down the blood vessels. If the placenta has NOT been delivered within an hour it is essential for you somehow to get the mother to a hospital.

10 Do not cut the cord if there is any hope of the doctor or midwife arriving shortly. If there is no such hope and the placenta has been delivered, or the cord has stopped pulsating, or more than 10 minutes has elapsed since the baby was born, then tie the cord firmly in 2 places with the sterilized string, about 50 mm (2 in) apart and about 150 mm (6 in) from the baby's navel. Make a back-up knot behind each of these and cut the cord between the two sets of ties. If a sterile dressing is available, put it over the cut end of the cord at the baby's navel; otherwise, leave it alone.

11 Wash the mother, give her a clean nightdress and a sanitary towel. Make her a cup of tea.

1. When the top of the baby's head appears, tell the mother not to push. The baby is usually born head first, facing downwards.
2. Support his head in the palm of your hand but DO NOT PULL. The next contraction will deliver the shoulders, and then the rest of his body will slip quickly out.
3. Hold the baby head downwards, to allow fluid to drain from his mouth. REMEMBER newly born babies are wet and slippery so be careful not to let him slip through your fingers.
4. Do not pull the cord, but wait for the placenta to be delivered naturally. This usually takes about 10–15 minutes. Make sure you keep the placenta as the doctor will want to examine it.

CHILLING

Adults

The healthy adult can normally cope very well with even extreme cold. Our bodies can make heat to replace that lost to the environment and so maintain an even temperature. It is only after prolonged exposure to cold, wet or windy weather that more body heat may be lost than can easily be replaced, so that the overall body temperature drops. Babies and old people, however, become much more easily chilled; babies because they lose heat more readily; old people because they cannot make heat so efficiently and they may become dangerously chilled in conditions that most of us could easily tolerate.

The symptoms of an adult suffering from hypothermia are a general slowing down, both physically and mentally. He may start to act irrationally or become irritable so that his behaviour seems out of character. His speech may become slurred and he may have difficulty is seeing; he is also likely to stumble and have fits of shivering or cramp, and become increasingly drowsy. Eventually he will become unconscious with slow shallow breathing and a slow pulse rate. The signs of hypothermia may develop so gradually that they may not be noticed until there has been a considerable drop in body temperature.

1 Prevent loss of further body heat in any way you can. If you are out in the open, try to make some form of shelter as protection from further wind or rain, and make sure that the casualty lies on something to insulate him from the ground. If possible put him in warm dry clothes and a sleeping bag. Use your own body contact to give him warmth if necessary.

2 Give a warm drink.

3 Once you reach home or habitation, a healthy young adult can safely be warmed up quickly by putting him in a hot bath.

4 An old person, who may have suffered cold exposure simply from being in an unheated house, should be rewarmed *gradually*, by being taken into warm surroundings and wrapped in blankets. DON'T give hot water bottles or use electric blankets. DO give warm, sweet drinks or hot soup.

REMEMBER

If a baby is dangerously chilled his tummy will be cool to the touch. DON'T be misled if his face and hands are healthily pink.

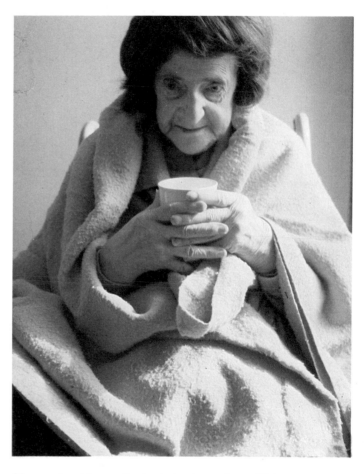

Above: In old age, the body becomes less efficient at making heat. Old people who have become chilled should be taken into a heated room and rewarmed gradually.

Babies

Because they lose heat so easily, new-born babies need to be kept very warm for the first weeks of life. A baby who is not quite warm enough will be fretful and listless. A baby who is becoming chilled will be quiet, and the skin of his chest and tummy will feel cold to the touch. Simply piling on extra clothes or blankets will not help – you need to warm his body first, by taking him into a warm room and giving a warm (not hot) drink. If the chilling has gone dangerously far the baby may be drowsy, floppy and unable to feed. In spite of the fact that he is so cold, his hands, feet and face may look bright pink. A baby in this condition needs immediate medical help and should be taken to hospital. If you cannot get him to hospital straight away, remove his clothes and get into a bed or sleeping-bag with him, so that you warm him gradually through skin-to-skin contact.

CHOKING

Any foreign body that lodges in the back of the throat or in the windpipe will cause choking. The most usual cause is food or drink 'going down the wrong way'. Usually these food particles are fairly small and do not block the airway completely, so that a certain amount of air can get past them, and the normal coughing and spluttering that the choking causes is enough to bring them back up again. Sometimes a larger piece of food, for example a chunk of meat, may completely obstruct the airway. This is known as the 'café coronary' because its most usual victim is the well-wined business-man who chokes on a piece of steak and whose companions, seeing him unable to breathe or speak, clutching his chest and turning blue-grey, assume that he has had a heart attack. This is often a fatal assumption because they then fail to give the appropriate first-aid, which would dislodge the obstruction and save him. For small children, who tend to put everything they can get hold of into their mouths, choking is an obvious hazard. Especially dangerous are smooth, round objects like marbles which may lodge in the windpipe and block it completely.

1 If the airway is not completely blocked, the person will be coughing and spluttering. If it is quite blocked, he will be unable even to cough, but will be struggling for breath and turning blue in the face. A series of sharp blows, delivered with the heel of the hand between the shoulder-blades, may be enough to dislodge the obstruction. Whenever possible, the person's head should be lower than his chest, e.g. by semi-suspending him over the edge of a table or chair.

2 If this does not work, try to hook out the obstruction from the back of the throat with a finger.

3 If you cannot dislodge the blockage, you must get the person to the hospital straight away.

4 If you do manage to dislodge the obstruction, the person may already have stopped breathing. You will need to carry out ARTIFICIAL RESPIRATION (p. 70).

SMALL CHILDREN

1 An infant who is choking should be held upside down by his ankles while you smack his back.

2 A child should be tipped forward over your knee so that his head and chest are lower than his hips. Slap him smartly on the back between the shoulder-blades.

3 If this does not work, try to hook the obstruction from the back of the throat with a finger.

HEIMLICH MANOEUVRE

This is a method for dealing with a complete obstruction of the windpipe which, although popular in America, is not yet widely used or recommended in this country. The technique is to give the abdomen a sudden and violent squeeze so that the diaphragm, and the air pressure inside the chest, are suddenly raised, shooting out the blockage, rather like a cork from a bottle. Some doctors feel that the method carries a risk of breaking a rib or causing even more serious internal injuries and that it is, anyway, not so effective as a series of sharp blows on the back. If the windpipe is completely blocked, and blows on the back fail to work, this may be the only chance to save a life.

1 Stand behind the person, putting both arms around him.

2 Place your hands one on top of the other in the centre of the chest just below the rib-cage and just above the navel.

3 Make the bottom hand into a fist.

4 Squeeze as hard as you can, with a slight upward pressure.

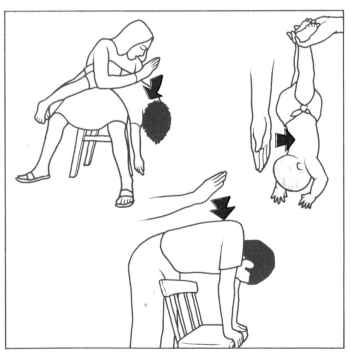

An obstruction in the throat can usually be dislodged by slapping the patient smartly on the back, between the shoulder-blades. Hold an infant head downwards by his feet, or lay an older child over your knees while you do this. An adult should try to get his head lower than his chest by hanging over the edge of a table or chair.

CONVULSIONS

Adults

Convulsions, although they are frightening for the onlooker who sees them for the first time, are not a medical emergency. First aid consists simply of making sure that the casualty does not endanger himself during the fit, and that his airway is kept clear while he is unconscious. Contrary to popular belief, not everyone bites his tongue during a fit and there is no need to stick corks, handkerchiefs or anything else between his teeth to prevent him doing so.

Major epilepsy (grand mal) is the most common cause of convulsions in adults, but convulsions may also be a sign of some other underlying disorder of the brain, e.g. following a head injury. They may also occur as a side effect of some drugs, or as a result of suddenly stopping a tranquillizing drug such as diazepam.

Occasionally people who experience major seizures with convulsions have some sort of warning, or 'aura' – they may feel strange, restless or irritable just before the convulsion. This may give them time to take preventive measures but they soon lose consciousness and fall, sometimes hurting themselves severely. At first they are in a state of rigidity, unable to breathe, their faces livid, the veins in their neck swollen and the eyes open and turned to one side. They then pass into a convulsive state with spasmodic contraction and relaxation of all the muscles of the body. Blood-stained froth may escape from the mouth. Control of both bladder and bowels may be lost so they may wet or soil themselves during the fit. Usually the fit lasts only a few minutes, then the muscles relax and the patient either regains consciousness, feeling dazed and confused, or falls into a deep sleep. When he wakes he will remember little or nothing about the fit.

1 Don't try to hold the person down, or to stop him jerking or thrashing about. Only restrain him if it is necessary to protect him from danger, particularly if he is likely to injure himself on any furniture, or is near a fire, for example. Undo tight clothing.

2 As soon as he becomes relaxed, wipe the froth from his mouth and place him in the RECOVERY POSITION (p. 72). Make sure that any vomit is cleared from his mouth and does not obstruct his breathing.

3 When he regains consciousness arrange for him to have clean dry clothes if he has wet or soiled himself. If he has bitten his tongue give him a mouth-wash and if he has cut himself during the fit, treat the cuts (see p. 50). Check for other injuries incurred during the fall.

4 If this is the patient's first fit, a doctor should be consulted so that the underlying cause can be discovered.

Children

Children are more 'convulsion-prone' than adults. Convulsions in an infant or small child, as with an adult, may be a sign of some underlying disorder such as epilepsy or brain disease. The most common type of convulsion in a small child is the 'febrile convulsion' which sometimes occurs when the child's temperature rises suddenly and rapidly, as often happens at the start of an infectious illness. Febrile convulsions tend to run in families, to be more usual in boys and to be most common between the ages of one and three. Many children grow out of them after the age of five. If your child has a fit for the first time you should always summon a doctor and ANY convulsion in a child that lasts longer than 2–3 minutes is a MEDICAL EMERGENCY.

Don't worry about a rise in temperature unless you know that your child is convulsion-prone. The body's built-in thermostat normally prevents an extreme rise in temperature. It is only under exceptional conditions, such as HEATSTROKE (p. 59), that fever may reach a dangerous level.

1 The most important thing is to stay with the child until the fit is over to make sure he does not injure himself. Try to put him on to something safe and soft if you can, like a wide bed, or a rug on the floor.

2 Don't try to restrain him, but do try to turn him so that he lies on his side or his front, with his head turned to one side, so that if he should vomit he will not inhale the vomit and choke.

3 Contact your doctor as soon as the child is calm again, or has fallen asleep.

4 If the child has a high temperature, cool him down as soon as you can. Take off his clothes and sponge him with tepid water, letting it dry on the skin.

OLD WIVES' TALE

Convulsions are NOT caused by:
Teething, Constipation or Thread Worms

PREVENTING CONVULSIONS

If your child has a tendency to febrile convulsions, your doctor will probably advise you to try to keep his temperature as low as you can next time he is ill. Take off all heavy bedclothes so that he is just covered by a sheet and one blanket, and make sure that his room is fairly cool. If his temperature rises above 103°F (39·4°C), take off his pyjamas and sponge him down with tepid water until it has fallen at least to 102°F. Junior aspirin will also help to keep the temperature down.

CRAMP

The sudden, painful muscle contractions of cramp can be caused by loss of salt and body fluids (either because you have been sweating a lot, or had a severe attack of diarrhoea or vomiting), or by chilling, as sometimes happens when you are swimming, or simply by poor circulation. Cramp most often strikes at night, usually in the calf and toe muscles, and old people may be particularly affected. There are a number of home remedies for cramp prevention, like raising the bottom of the bed, for example, but none of them can really be guaranteed to work. Wherever the cramp is, the treatment is the same – stretch the muscle as hard as you can, by straightening it from its cramped position, and massage it. If the cramp has been caused by loss of body fluids or salt, drink slightly salted water – about half a teaspoon of salt to half a litre of water will replace the salt and fluid without tasting too unpleasant.

If the cramp is in the calf, stand on that leg, straightening the knee and forcing your heel down on the floor. If the toes are curled in by cramp, straighten them by pressing upwards, or standing on the ball of your foot. If the fingers are affected uncurl them and massage them well.

CUTS & GRAZES

Small cuts with slight bleeding need very little treatment. The bleeding will stop of its own accord as the blood clots. If blood is flowing freely, press gently but firmly on the wound with a cotton wool or gauze pad – or with any clean material – for about two minutes. Heavier bleeding may take longer to stop. If, after you have applied pressure for four minutes it still has not lessened, consult a doctor. The cut may be bad enough to need stitching. If blood *spurts* from the wound, or flows so heavily that you cannot lessen the flow, see SERIOUS BLEEDING (p. 36). Any wound which is very large and dirty should be shown to a doctor – you may need an anti-tetanus injection.

Bleeding will carry most of the dirt and germs out of the wound. Gently wiping it, from the inside out, with swabs of cotton wool (using a fresh swab for each stroke) will make sure that it is quite clean and help reduce the risk of infection. Soak cotton wool swabs in an antiseptic solution. Hydrogen peroxide B.P., which can be used straight from the bottle, is the easiest. If you use any other antiseptic solution, make sure you follow the directions for dilution which are printed on the bottle – too strong a solution will damage the tissues and do more harm than good. If you have no antiseptic at all, use plain soap and water to wash around the wound. A small wound may not need a dressing and will probably heal more quickly if you keep it dry and let the air get at it.

Cuts on the fingers, even if small, can be particularly painful because they tend to 'catch' on things and are liable to become infected. Keep them covered with a dry adhesive plaster for 24 hours or until they begin to heal.

If the cut is large enough to gape but is not very deep, or if it is on a finger or knee so that bending the joint makes the edges open, draw the edges together so that they just meet, and put one or two strips of a porous synthetic surgical tape across the cut. If the cut gapes so badly that you cannot hold its edges together like this, it probably needs stitching and you should consult a doctor. A deep or jagged cut, and any cut on the face, unless it is very superficial, should also be shown to a doctor. Even trivial cuts on the face are often better stitched, as this helps them to heal with as little scarring as possible.

GRAZES

Although they are usually trivial, grazes can be very painful because a relatively large area of the outermost layer of skin, which contains the pain-sensitive nerve endings, is damaged. If there is visible grit on the graze remove what you can with a swab of wet cotton wool. Swab from the centre of the wound outwards. Cover the graze with a piece of dry gauze until the scab has started to form.

Below: To clean a cut or graze, always swab away from the wound. If grit or dirt is embedded beneath the skin, it should be properly cleaned and dressed by a doctor.

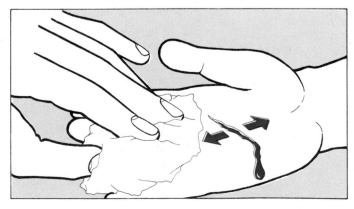

ACTION CHECK

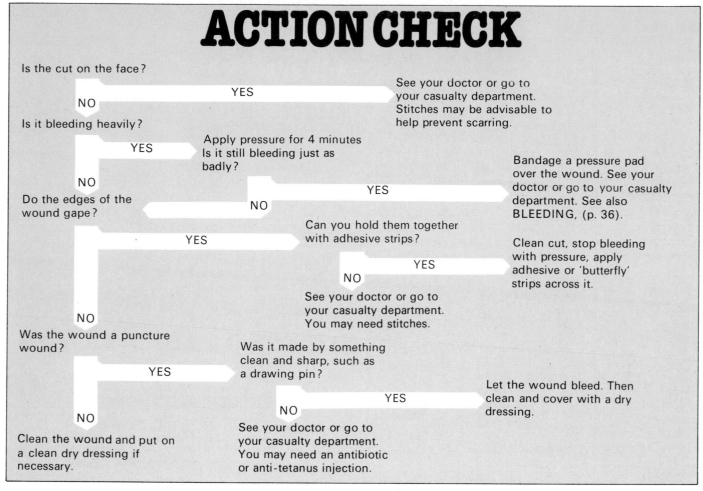

HEALING

Minor cuts and grazes should heal quite quickly, in about a week to a fortnight, depending on the size of the cut and its whereabouts. At first you will see a clear, yellowish fluid in the wound. This is serum, which later forms the scab. The edges of the would will be pink or red during the healing process. If you can see thick, yellowish-white pus in the wound, or if it becomes very red, swollen or tender, it has become infected and you should consult your doctor.

1 Make sure the wound is clean, using an antiseptic solution or plain soap and water to clean around it.

2 If possible, leave it uncovered, unless it is likely to become dirty and infected.

3 If the wound gapes, hold the edges together with surgical tape.

4 If the wound becomes infected, is deep, jagged or on the face, see a doctor.

PUNCTURE WOUNDS

The special danger of a wound made by something like a nail, or a tin-tack, is that although it may look tiny and bleed very little, dirt can be carried deep into the body and the wound may become infected. *Never* try to stop a puncture wound bleeding – bleeding is the most effective way of cleaning it. When the bleeding stops of its own accord wash the wound and put a clean dry dressing over it. If the object that caused the wound was quite clean there is no need to see a doctor, although you should keep a careful check on the wound for the following few days just to make sure that it does not become infected. If the wound was caused by anything dirty, by stepping on a rusty nail for example, you should see a doctor. He may feel that you should have an antibiotic or an anti-tetanus injection. This also applies to any cuts or grazes received on agricultural limb following a wound, consult your doctor.

Another danger of a deep cut or puncture wound is that underlying nerves or tendons may be damaged. If you notice any numbness, tingling or weakness in a limb following a wound, consult your doctor.

STAB WOUNDS

A stab wound may penetrate the chest wall so that air bubbles in and out of it as the patient breathes. Blood or blood-stained bubbles may also come from the wound, as the patient breathes out. Cover the wound with an airtight seal by strapping a pad, sheet of plastic or metal foil over it. Lie the patient down, but with his head and shoulders raised, and leaning towards the injured side.

DIABETIC EMERGENCY

Diabetes mellitus (sugar diabetes) is a disease in which the body is unable to absorb sugar, because of a lack of a substance called insulin. The diabetic has to take regular doses of insulin to keep the sugar in his blood at the right level. If he misses a meal or uses up more sugar than he realizes, or overinjects himself with insulin, there will be too much 'loose' insulin in his body. He will rapidly become confused, shocked, and lose consciousness; this is an *insulin coma*.

Too little insulin may lead to a different kind of coma, called a *diabetic coma*, in which the casualty will look flushed, his skin will be dry and his breath will have a characteristic smell, similar to nail varnish.

If you are dealing with a known diabetic who is faint or unconscious, he is much more likely to be in an insulin coma rather than a diabetic coma, because the latter has a very gradual onset.

1 If the patient is conscious, give him something sugary such as a drink with two tablespoonfuls of sugar, or lumps of sugar. If, however, it is obvious that the patient is going into a diabetic coma, e.g. by the smell of his breath, then sugary drinks, sugarlumps, etc. should *not* be given.

2 Place him in the RECOVERY POSITION (p. 72) and summon medical help.

DIFFICULTY IN BREATHING (ASTHMA)

Breathing out is usually a passive and effortless procedure. The lung tissue is stretched when we breathe in, and the natural elasticity of the lungs then drives the air out. Sometimes the breathing tubes (or bronchioles) become constricted so that you cannot breathe out naturally but have to use your chest muscles to force the air out. Spells of this forced, wheezy and difficult breathing are called asthma. Asthma is often an allergic condition, but can also be the result of some form of heart trouble or be due to an infection such as bronchitis. Attacks of asthma usually occur suddenly and at night.

1 Sit the patient up in a comfortable position. It is easier to use the 'extra' chest muscles for breathing if sitting and leaning slightly forward. Loosen tight clothing and ensure a liberal supply of fresh air.

2 Reassure him. The inability to release a breath in order to take another one is frightening and may make him feel panic-stricken.

3 If this is a first attack, call a doctor straight away. If asthma attacks happen regularly, your doctor will tell you how to deal with them.

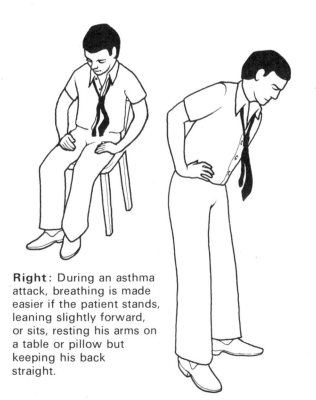

Right: During an asthma attack, breathing is made easier if the patient stands, leaning slightly forward, or sits, resting his arms on a table or pillow but keeping his back straight.

DROWNING

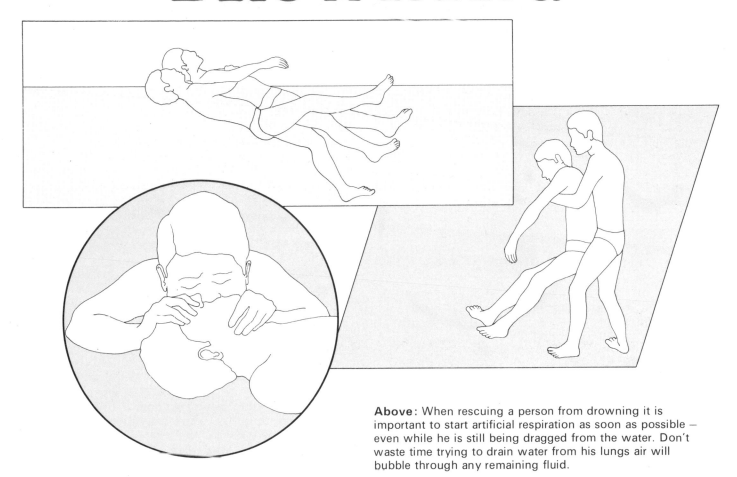

Above: When rescuing a person from drowning it is important to start artificial respiration as soon as possible — even while he is still being dragged from the water. Don't waste time trying to drain water from his lungs air will bubble through any remaining fluid.

When rescuing a drowning person, DON'T jump in after him if you are a weak swimmer or a non-swimmer yourself. Instead, try to find a rope or life-belt to throw to him, to keep him afloat until you can get help. If you are in a boat, switch off the engine before you get too close. Pull the person in over the stern, not the side of the boat, or you may capsize it. Should the boat capsize, STAY WITH IT. Swimming will make you lose body heat and in many water-accidents such heat loss can be as great a danger as that of drowning. The boat will support you and make you easier for a potential rescuer to see.

1 If the person is coughing, choking or vomiting when he is brought out of the water, he must still be breathing, and therefore you do not need to begin resuscitation. Immediately place him face downwards in the RECOVERY POSITION (p. 72), so that fluid can drain from his mouth and lungs.

2 If he is unconscious and not breathing, DON'T WASTE TIME trying to get water out of his lungs before you start giving mouth-to-mouth resuscitation. Some water left in the lungs is unimportant and will eventually be absorbed or ejected. What matters most is to get him breathing again.

3 Take special care to clear the airway before you begin resuscitation. It may be blocked by seaweed, sand or vomit.

4 Start resuscitation as soon as you can – even while he is still being carried from the water if this is possible. The longer the delay in getting air through to his lungs, the less chance there is of a full recovery. See MOUTH-TO-MOUTH RESUSCITATION (p. 70).

5 Continue resuscitation until help arrives, or until he starts to breathe again.

6 Once he is breathing, make sure that he is not chilled. HYPOTHERMIA (p. 47) may result from even a short period of immersion in cold water.

DON'T
Don't waste time. If someone else is there to help, you can start giving artificial respiration as the casualty is being carried from the water. DON'T try to force water out of the lungs. You may cause internal injury. DON'T give up hope. Continue artificial respiration until help arrives.

ELECTRIC SHOCK

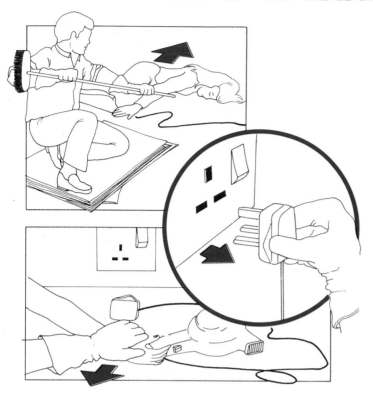

Above: If you can't turn the power off, stand on a thick layer of newspapers and break the electrical contact using a wooden broom-handle or other non-conducting object to push or pull the person clear.

How dangerous an electric shock can be depends on both the voltage and the current that passes across your heart. In Europe, the normal domestic voltage is 200–250 volts. This can kill under special circumstances, if there is very good electrical contact between the power source, the person touching it and the ground. In America the normal voltage is 110 volts which is very much safer although again, in some special circumstances, it can be lethal. Some factories have higher voltage supplies of approximately 440 volts and this sort of power source is extremely dangerous. Highest of all are the voltages used by the electricity supply industry. Special equipment is needed to handle these. On no account should you try to rescue anyone who is in contact with such a high voltage source.

If you touch a defective electrical appliance in which a live wire inside is touching the casing, so that the casing itself is live, you will probably get only a very mild shock, provided your hands are dry and you are standing on a dry floor. Water is a good conductor of electricity. If you touch a faulty appliance with wet hands or while standing on a wet bathroom floor, the shock will be much worse. If you touch a faulty electrical appliance while you are actually in your bath, it will kill you. This is why it is illegal to have power points in a bathroom. While a small child might get

away with poking a matchstick into the 'live' hole of a power socket, because wood is a bad conductor of electricity, doing the same thing with a piece of wire or his finger would result in a very nasty shock indeed.

A mild electric shock will merely produce a brief 'pins and needles' sensation. A severe shock makes the muscles contract, so that someone who has touched a live object may have his hand clenched around it. A bad electric shock can render you unconscious and stop both breathing and heart beat.

An electric current can also burn (see p. 43). Any electrical burn should be shown to a doctor. Although it may look small it is possible it may be quite deep.

1 Switch off the current at the mains, or pull out the plug. Until this has been done DON'T TOUCH the casualty – you will only get a shock yourself.

2 If you cannot switch off the current, break the electrical contact by dragging the person away from it. But before doing so, stand on some dry, non-conducting material (wood, rubber, dry cloth, layers of newspaper) and try to push him away with whatever non-conducting object you can find. If this is not possible, you can drag him away providing you insulate your hand as thickly as you can, either by wearing rubber gloves, wrapping your hand in dry cloth or newspaper, or even by using a pair of rubber-soled shoes or Wellington boots. In many cases it may be easier to push the contact, e.g. defective appliance, away from the person with a broom-handle.

3 If the person is unconscious, watch for signs that his heart may have stopped. He may look very pale and blue around the lips. If you lift his eyelids, his pupils will be enlarged. Feel for the carotid pulse at either side of the neck – if you cannot feel it start EXTERNAL CARDIAC MASSAGE if you have been trained in this technique (p. 74).

4 Check his breathing. If he is not breathing start ARTIFICIAL RESPIRATION (p. 70).

5 If he is breathing but unconscious, place him in the RECOVERY POSITION (p. 72).

6 Telephone for an ambulance or doctor.

DON'T
Don't touch a person who has received an electric shock until the power has been turned off.

FAINTING

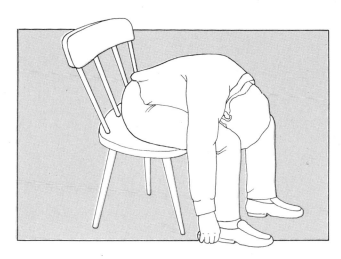

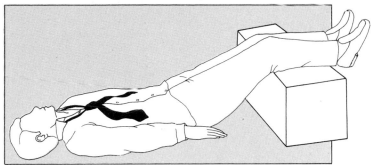

Above: If the fainting patient is breathing normally, lie him on his back with his feet raised; loosen any tight clothing.
Left: If he is feeling faint, loosen tight clothing and make him sit with his head between his knees.

Fainting is caused by a temporary lack of blood supply to the brain. This can happen if you stand up suddenly after stooping or lying down or when you first get up after a long period of convalescence or bed-rest. You may also feel faint if you have been standing very still for a long time. Fainting can also be a form of nervous shock following an emotional upset or severe injury or pain.

If you just *feel* faint – turning pale, sweating, feeling dizzy, lightheaded or unsteady – you will probably be able to stop yourself fainting by immediately lying down, or sitting with your head forwards between your knees. Loosen any tight clothing and breathe deeply. Flex the muscles of your legs, thighs and buttocks.

A true faint is a brief loss of consciousness.

If you see someone faint, take the following action:

1 Lie the patient down, raising his legs so that they are above the level of his head.

2 Loosen any tight clothing at neck or waist, and see that he has plenty of fresh air.

3 If he has any difficulty in breathing, place him in the RECOVERY POSITION (p. 72).

4 As he regains consciousness, colour should return to his skin. Sit him up and give him small sips of water. When he has quite recovered, offer him a cup of sweetened tea or coffee, but only *if you are sure* the faint was not the result of any injury or severe pain. Don't give a glass of brandy or anything alcoholic.

A normal faint needs no further treatment. If recovery is not complete within half an hour, call your doctor. There may be some underlying cause of the faint that needs treatment.

FINGER & TOE INJURIES

If you drop a heavy object on your toe, or trap a finger in a door, the injury is likely to be extremely painful. Even if the skin is not broken there may be bleeding under the nail. Put the finger (or toe) under a running cold water tap for two minutes. This will help to reduce any bleeding. Then see your doctor. He will, if necessary, make a tiny hole in the nail to release the blood; this will release the pressure on the nail and reduce the pain. If this is not done, and if the growing nail-bed is damaged by the blow, the nail may become loose and finally drop off. If the nail does begin to shed, put adhesive plaster over it and let the new nail push the old one off gradually as it grows. If you do this, the new nail is less likely to be misshapen.

See also CUTS AND GRAZES (p. 50).

FISH HOOKS

Fish hooks embedded in the skin as the result of inaccurate casting are best dealt with by a doctor but, in an emergency, they can, if not too large or deeply embedded, be removed with the aid of a pair of wire clippers or pliers.

1 Don't try to pull out a fish hook which has pierced the skin – because it is barbed it will tear the flesh.

2 Push the hook gently through the skin until the barb is free, then cut off the barb. You should then be able to draw the hook *back* through the skin.

3 If it seems easier, the *shank* can be cut off close to the skin once you have pushed the barb through clear of the skin. Then you can push the hook on through.

4 Clean the wound thoroughly with soap and water and watch carefully over the next few days for signs of infection.

5 If the hook is large, push it through till the barb is clear of the skin, and then tape it to the skin until you can reach a doctor.

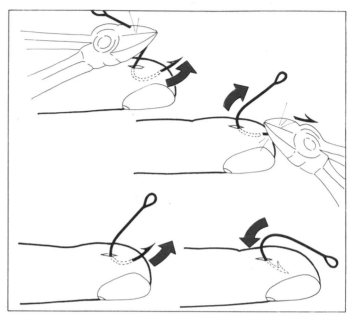

Above: Remove a barbed fish hook by pushing it through, then either clipping off the end and withdrawing the hook, or clipping the shank and pushing it through.

FOREIGN BODIES

IN THE EARS

Children are quite likely to put small objects – usually small round objects that are difficult to remove – into their ears. If you can see the object, and if you can get hold of it with a pair of tweezers, you may be able to lift it out. If you cannot see it, DON'T POKE ABOUT.

It is said that insects occasionally fly into ears, though the chances of this happening must be very small. However, they do creep into them, e.g. earwigs whilst camping. If this happens pour drops of lukewarm olive oil into the ear, pulling the ear lobe backwards as you do so, to straighten the ear canal. Keep the head tilted to the opposite side for a few minutes then let the oil run out. With luck, the insect will come out with it.

IN THE EYES

Very often the natural reactions of tears and blinking which an eyelash or a piece of dust in the eye produce are enough to wash the foreign body out. If not, examine the eye in a good light. If you can see the object, you may be able to remove it yourself, *provided* that it is on the *white part* of the eye. This part is fairly tough and

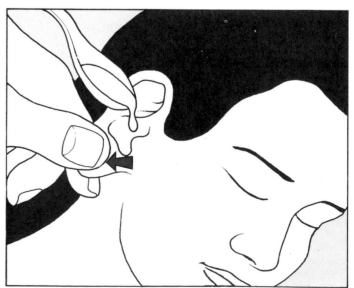

Above: Float out an insect which is trapped in an ear by dropping warmed oil into the ear from a spoon. Keep the head on one side for a few minutes, then let the oil run out.

will not be easily damaged by gentle attempts to remove the foreign body, but the transparent cornea, with the coloured iris set under it, is much more delicate and easily scratched. Anything lying on this part of the eye, OR anything which is actually *embedded* in any part of the eye, should be removed by a doctor as quickly as possible. If your eye is struck by a flying particle while you are using a power saw or drilling metal, consult your doctor anyway. The particles may hit the eyeball with such force that they become embedded in it.

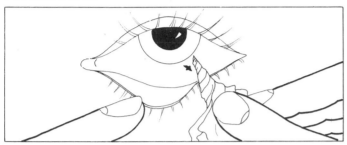

Above: A foreign body easily visible on the white of the eye can usually be removed with the corner of a clean handkerchief, or a piece of damp, twisted cotton wool.

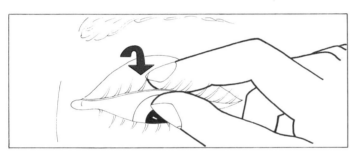

Above: A foreign body under an upper eyelid may be removed by drawing the upper lid gently outwards and down over the lower lid.

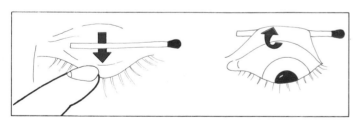

Above: You may be able to see and remove a foreign body trapped under the upper eyelid by pulling the lid up and outwards over a matchstick pressed gently against it. Remove it with the corner of a clean handkerchief or a piece of damp, twisted cotton wool, as in the top picture.

1 Wash the eye out in water or (better still) in a weak salt solution – one teaspoon of salt per pint of boiled water which *has been allowed to cool*. Ask the casualty to blink a few times under water.

2 If this fails pull down the lower lid. If you can see the foreign body on the white of the eye, try to lift it off with the corner of a clean handkerchief, or a damp twist of cotton wool.

3 If the foreign body feels as though it is under the upper lid, tell the person to look down, then gently draw the upper lid down over the lower one.

4 If this fails and if you cannot easily get the person to a doctor, you may be able to turn the upper lid 'inside out' over a matchstick to help you get at whatever lies underneath it. Stand behind the casualty, so that his head is resting on your chest and ask him to look down. Place a matchstick just above the eyelashes on the top lid and press it gently backwards. Then, taking hold of the eyelashes, turn the lid backwards over the match.

5 If the eye still feels gritty or painful, OR if the object is anywhere but on the white of the eye, OR, if it is embedded in any part of the eye, cover the eye with a pad of cotton wool, anchored with adhesive tape, and take the casualty to your doctor. If the eye pad is uncomfortable, wear dark glasses instead.

6 NEVER RUB AN INJURED EYE.

Chemicals in the eye

Any acid or alkaline material, such as ammonia, bleach, household cleaners or lime, can damage the eye very quickly if accidentally splashed into it.

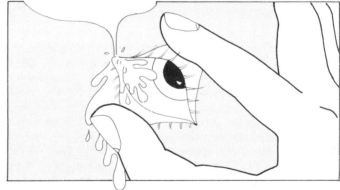

Above: Flush out corrosive fluid splashed in the eye with running water.

Wash the eye out IMMEDIATELY. If possible get the casualty to immerse his whole face in water and blink his eye repeatedly, or gently pour water over the injured eye from a jug, holding the eyelids apart and inclining the head so that the contaminated water runs straight off the face and cannot splash into the other eye. Take the patient to the hospital casualty department.

OBJECTS IN THE NOSE

Do not try to remove an object stuck in a child's nose. Ensure that he does not touch his nose and that he breathes through his mouth. Persuade him not to sniff or inhale through his nose. Take him to your doctor who will have the right sort of instruments to extract the object.

HEAD INJURIES

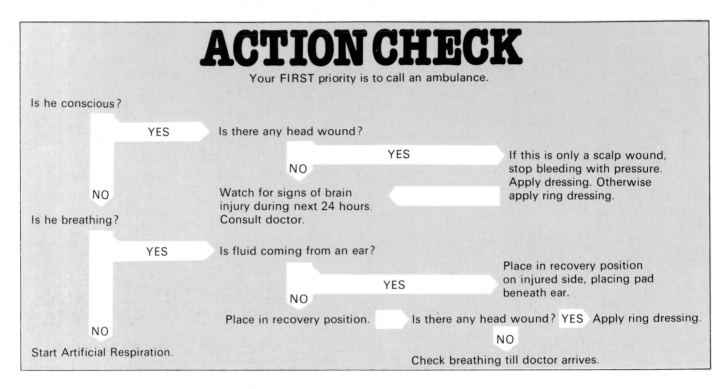

ACTION CHECK

Your FIRST priority is to call an ambulance.

Is he conscious?

→ YES → Is there any head wound?

→ YES → If this is only a scalp wound, stop bleeding with pressure. Apply dressing. Otherwise apply ring dressing.

NO → Watch for signs of brain injury during next 24 hours. Consult doctor.

NO →

Is he breathing?

→ YES → Is fluid coming from an ear?

→ YES → Place in recovery position on injured side, placing pad beneath ear.

NO → Place in recovery position. → Is there any head wound? YES Apply ring dressing.

NO → Check breathing till doctor arrives.

NO → Start Artificial Respiration.

A blow to the head does not necessarily damage the brain, even if the skull is fractured. A crack in the skull will heal just like any other fractured bone BUT a 'depressed' fracture, that is, one in which the bone presses inwards on to the brain, is serious and may produce symptoms of a brain injury (p. 59). Sometimes a blow to the jaw or even a heavy fall on the feet or on to the base of the spine can fracture the floor of the skull. If you see straw-coloured or blood-stained fluid coming from the ear or nose or from a bloodshot eye after this kind of fall, it suggests that the base of the skull has been fractured.

A severe jolt or bang on the head, even if it does not damage the skull itself, may sometimes 'shake up' the brain so that it knocks against the inside of the skull, causing the temporary loss of consciousness called *concussion*. Someone who is concussed will be unconscious, or at least extremely dazed, for a short time, perhaps only a few seconds, and is likely to feel sick or vomit as he recovers. He may not remember anything that happened just before or after the accident. Occasionally the injury causing the concussion may be more serious than it seems, because a blood vessel inside the skull has been damaged, so that a blood clot forms inside the skull pressing on the brain. If this condition of 'compression' develops, the patient's face will become flushed, his breathing noisy, his pulse slow, and his pupils may be unequal in size. Someone who has been concussed playing football, for example, may go on playing, apparently quite normally, and only

later develop signs of brain injury. So you should always keep a careful watch for the next 24 hours on anyone who has had a blow to the head or a short period of concussion; anyone who has been unconscious should be seen by a doctor before starting work or taking up any other activities again.

1 Telephone for an ambulance.

2 If the casualty is unconscious, place him in the RECOVERY POSITION (p. 72), but see POSSIBLE SPINAL INJURY (p. 59). If you can see fluid coming from an ear, put a pad over the ear and turn the person on to the injured side so that fluid can drain from it.

3 Check the breathing – you may need to start ARTIFICIAL RESPIRATION (p. 70).

4 Once you have placed the casualty in the recovery position, deal with any wounds. If there is bleeding from a head wound do not try to stop it with direct pressure in case there is an underlying skull fracture. Instead, put on a ring dressing, with a bandage over it, so that there is pressure around the wound, but not on it (p. 37).

5 If the casualty is unconscious, or if he recovers consciousness after a short period, make him rest and watch him carefully for the next few hours for any signs of brain injury. *Make sure he sees a doctor* before he returns to work or continues whatever he was doing.

SYMPTOMS OF BRAIN INJURY

Unconsciousness
There may be immediate loss of consciousness after the injury or unconsciousness may follow a period of extreme drowsiness.

Noisy breathing

Flushed face
(because the body temperature is likely to rise)

Slow pulse

Twitching of the limbs

Convulsions

Abnormal pupils
Either unequal in size, both dilated, or unresponsive (that is, not contracting) when a light is shone on them.

Muscle weakness or paralysis

POSSIBLE SPINAL INJURY

If you think there is a chance that the spine may have been damaged, perhaps by a heavy or awkward fall, DON'T move or place the casualty in the recovery position. Make sure that the head is turned to one side, however, so that, if the casualty vomits, he will not choke.

HEAD INJURIES AND CONCUSSION

Always tell your doctor straight away if any of the following symptoms develops after a head injury.

● Increasing severe headache

● Continuous vomiting

● Double vision

● Unnatural drowsiness

● Unconsciousness

HEAT EXHAUSTION & HEATSTROKE

Very hot weather – or any other hot conditions – may, especially if you are not used to them, make you feel sick, giddy and listless. You may have a headache and your skin will feel damp. This condition is known as *heat exhaustion* and it is caused by the body's efforts to keep cool by opening up small blood vessels in the skin so that more blood can be diverted to the surface of the body. Because so much blood accumulates in the skin, less is available to be pumped around the rest of the body. The blood supply to the brain is decreased and it is this that causes the feeling of faintness, sometimes even actual fainting, which you may experience. You can prevent heat exhaustion by giving yourself time to get acclimatized to extra hot weather conditions, if you go on holiday, by keeping in the shade as much as possible at first, drinking plenty of fluids (though not alcohol) and taking extra salt. If you do start to feel sick or giddy, rest in a cool room and drink as much fluid as you can. A solution of half a teaspoonful of salt to half a litre of water will help to replace the fluid and salt lost in perspiration. Salt loss may be indicated by severe muscle cramps.

If the sun is very hot and you are in it for a long time, particularly if you over-exert yourself, your body may no longer be able to control its temperature by sweating. Your temperature will begin to rise, usually quite suddenly, and you will develop the more serious condition of *heatstroke*. You may have a temperature of 40°C (104°F) or even higher, your skin will be flushed and dry and you may vomit and lose consciousness. If conscious, you will probably have a headache and feel dizzy.

1 The purpose of the treatment is to bring the temperature down as quickly as possible. Strip the patient and wrap him in a cold wet sheet. A child may be put straight into a bath of cold water, and sponged.

2 If he is unconscious, place him in the RECOVERY POSITION (p. 72).

3 Fan him, either by hand or using an electric fan or a hair dryer set to 'cold'. This will help to cool him down even more quickly.

4 Take his temperature every few minutes. Once his temperature has been lowered to 101°F (38°C), replace the wet sheet with a dry one, but keep him in a cool room, and make sure his temperature does not start to rise again. If it does, repeat the wet sheet treatment.

5 Anyone who has suffered heatstroke should be sent to hospital urgently, or seen by a doctor as soon as possible.

HEART ATTACK

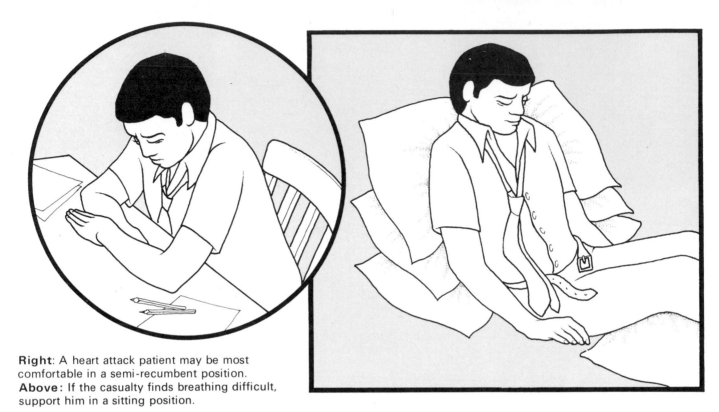

Right: A heart attack patient may be most comfortable in a semi-recumbent position.
Above: If the casualty finds breathing difficult, support him in a sitting position.

When the blood supply is cut off from part of the heart muscle there is usually, though not always, a gripping pain in the chest that often radiates to the left shoulder or arm, and may spread to the throat and jaw as well. Someone who has suffered a heart attack may also be SHOCKED (p. 69), so that he is pale, weak and faint with cold clammy skin. He may be blue around the lips and have difficulty in breathing. If the attack is severe, he may lose consciousness.

If someone has a severe chest pain that is brought on by exercise but gets better when he rests it is probably *angina*. A severe chest pain that does not disappear after the person has been resting for a few minutes *may* be a heart attack. The first time you, or anyone else, has such a pain you should treat it as a medical emergency and call a doctor straight away.

1 Telephone for an ambulance or for the doctor.

2 Move the patient as little as possible. The more he remains still, the less work his heart will have to do.

3 Make him as comfortable as you can without moving him unnecessarily. If the patient sat down in a chair when he felt the attack, there is no need to move him. If he is lying on the floor or on a bed he will probably be most comfortable with his head and shoulders propped up on a couple of pillows.

4 Loosen any tight clothing at neck, chest or waist.

5 If he finds breathing difficult, prop him up in a sitting position.

6 The patient is probably shocked. Keep him warm by covering with a coat. Don't give a hot water bottle.

7 If he becomes unconscious, place him in the RECOVERY POSITION (p. 72) and check breathing and pulse at regular intervals.

8 If breathing fails, start ARTIFICIAL RESPIRATION (p. 70).

9 If the heart stops start EXTERNAL CARDIAC MASSAGE if you have been trained in this technique (p. 74).

10 People who suffer from angina usually carry tablets of glyceryl trinitrate or glass capsules of amyl nitrate. Either of these will usually relieve the pain of angina attacks but they should not be given as treatment to anyone who has had a heart attack.

DON'T
Don't delay in calling the doctor. Assume that any severe chest pain, especially if it radiates down an arm, is a heart attack.

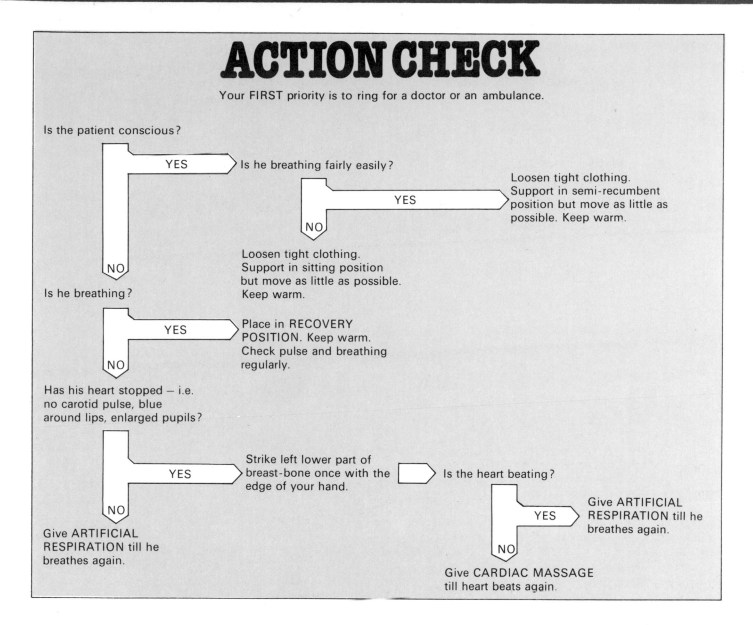

ACTION CHECK

Your FIRST priority is to ring for a doctor or an ambulance.

Is the patient conscious?

YES → Is he breathing fairly easily?

YES → Loosen tight clothing. Support in semi-recumbent position but move as little as possible. Keep warm.

NO → Loosen tight clothing. Support in sitting position but move as little as possible. Keep warm.

NO → Is he breathing?

YES → Place in RECOVERY POSITION. Keep warm. Check pulse and breathing regularly.

NO → Has his heart stopped — i.e. no carotid pulse, blue around lips, enlarged pupils?

YES → Strike left lower part of breast-bone once with the edge of your hand. → Is the heart beating?

YES → Give ARTIFICIAL RESPIRATION till he breathes again.

NO → Give CARDIAC MASSAGE till heart beats again.

NO → Give ARTIFICIAL RESPIRATION till he breathes again.

NOSEBLEEDS

Nose-bleeds may be the result of a blow on the nose, nose-picking, or too much nose-blowing during a cold or hay fever, but very often they happen spontaneously and for no apparent reason. Some people have repeated nose-bleeds, probably because the small blood vessels in the membrane that lines the nose are particularly fragile. Occasionally, if nose-bleeds are a real nuisance, a fragile blood vessel can be sealed off, or cauterized.

Lean forward over a bowl, pinching the nostrils firmly together. Keep this up for ten minutes. If the nosebleed hasn't stopped by then (and it most probably will have done), repeat the treatment. An ice-pack, or handkerchief wrung out in ice-cold water, placed on the bridge of the nose, may help. If it is still bleeding just as badly after half an hour, see a doctor. Don't blow the nose for some hours after the bleeding has stopped.

Children dislike the sight of their own blood. If a child's nose is bleeding heavily, get him to bend over a wash-basin while you hold his nostrils together and keep the tap running to wash the blood away.

If there is a discharge of clear, or blood-stained fluid from the nose after a head injury this may be because the base of the skull has been fractured. Allow the fluid to drain, and lie the patient on the injured side.

OLD WIVES' TALE

Nosebleeds are NOT caused by high blood pressure. People with high blood pressure can, of course, have nosebleeds, but they are no more likely to have them than anyone else.

POISONING

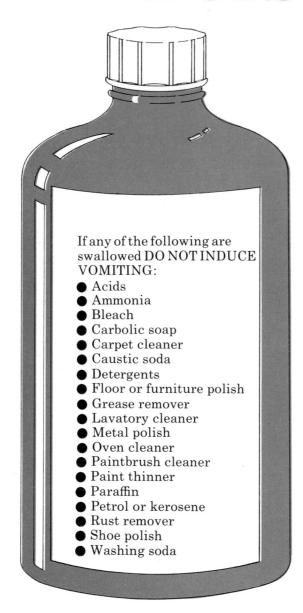

If any of the following are swallowed DO NOT INDUCE VOMITING:

- Acids
- Ammonia
- Bleach
- Carbolic soap
- Carpet cleaner
- Caustic soda
- Detergents
- Floor or furniture polish
- Grease remover
- Lavatory cleaner
- Metal polish
- Oven cleaner
- Paintbrush cleaner
- Paint thinner
- Paraffin
- Petrol or kerosene
- Rust remover
- Shoe polish
- Washing soda

Corrosive or burning substances, such as petrol, paraffin, household cleaners or paint strippers are especially hazardous. *If you know that this sort of substance has been swallowed*, NEVER *try to make the casualty sick* – the burning vomit will damage his throat and there is an even more serious risk of it being inhaled and damaging the lungs.

1 Telephone for an ambulance.

2 Try to find out what the poison is. If the casualty is conscious, ask him – if you leave it too long he may not be able to answer you.

3 If you know that a corrosive substance has been swallowed, or if you can see any signs of burning around lips and mouth that might indicate this, you must not try to make the casualty sick. Instead, *dilute* the poison so that it does less damage to the stomach, by giving one pint of tepid milk (or water if milk is not available), in sips. Gently sponge face and mouth to wash away any traces of the chemical remaining.

DON'T try to pour liquid into his mouth if he is unconscious – you may choke him.

4 If you are dealing with a conscious adult who has just swallowed a large quantity of pills, or with a conscious child who has just eaten something you think is poisonous, you may be able to rid the body of the poison by making him vomit.

NEVER GIVE EMETICS, E.G. SALT OR MUSTARD AND WATER.

Just put your fingers to the back of his throat and wriggle them until he vomits. If this doesn't work the first time, don't try again.

5 If you arrive on the scene some time after the poison has been taken, don't try to induce vomiting – the poison will already have begun to be absorbed into the body.

6 Keep any bottles of pills or medicines that may be lying near and, if the casualty has vomited, keep a sample of the vomit, too. Give these to the doctor or ambulance staff when they arrive.

7 Watch carefully to make sure the casualty does not lose consciousness. If he does, put him in the RECOVERY POSITION (p. 72) and check his breathing regularly. Many poisons affect the respiratory system; if breathing stops you will need to start ARTIFICIAL RESPIRATION (p. 70).

The victims of accidental poisoning are almost always children but adults (apart from deliberate self-poisoning) can eat contaminated food or poisonous mushrooms, inhale lethal gases without realizing it or even take a swig from a gin bottle that someone has used as a container for paint-cleaner or paraffin without relabelling it. Those who are elderly and absent-minded (or younger and drunk) may take accidental overdoses of sleeping pills or other drugs.

If a poison is swallowed it may cause vomiting, with stomach pains and diarrhoea. Immediate vomiting may mean that the body has rid itself of the poisonous substance. If the poison is absorbed into the blood, or inhaled, it can affect the nervous system, cause unconsciousness, failure of breathing and eventually death.

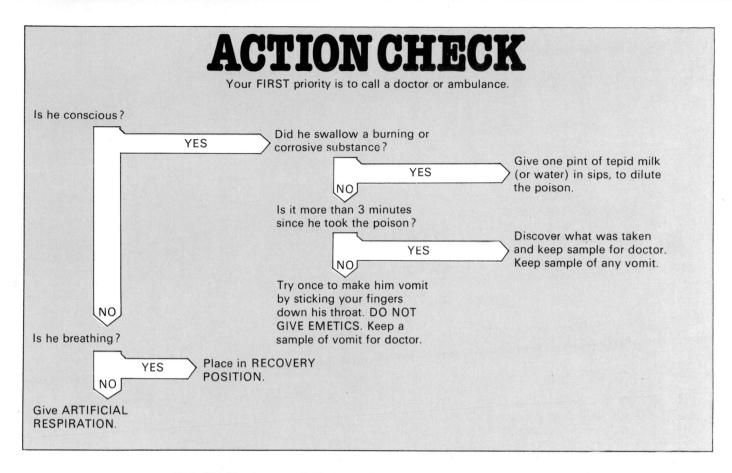

ACTION CHECK

Your FIRST priority is to call a doctor or ambulance.

Is he conscious?

YES → Did he swallow a burning or corrosive substance?

NO → **YES** → Give one pint of tepid milk (or water) in sips, to dilute the poison.

NO → Is it more than 3 minutes since he took the poison?

NO → **YES** → Discover what was taken and keep sample for doctor. Keep sample of any vomit.

NO → Try once to make him vomit by sticking your fingers down his throat. DO NOT GIVE EMETICS. Keep a sample of vomit for doctor.

NO → Is he breathing?

YES → Place in RECOVERY POSITION.

NO → Give ARTIFICIAL RESPIRATION.

SPLINTERS & THORNS

Splinters are among the most frequent mishaps, and although they seem almost too trivial to be called an injury, they can be extremely painful, so it is worth trying to remove them if you can. A small, obstinately buried one will probably do no harm if you leave it, gently wiping the skin around it with a solution of hydrogen peroxide. If the wound becomes infected – red, swollen, warm or tender – consult a doctor.

1 If no loose end is available, but you can see the splinter quite clearly, it is probably lying just below the surface of the skin. Sterilize a needle in a match flame and gently tear the skin a little way along the line of the splinter, starting at the point at which the splinter entered the skin. You may then be able to lift up the end of the splinter with the needle point and tweeze it out.

2 If the thorn or splinter has gone straight down into the skin, so that you can only see one end, continuous probing with a needle in an attempt to extract it will be painful. Most small splinters work their way

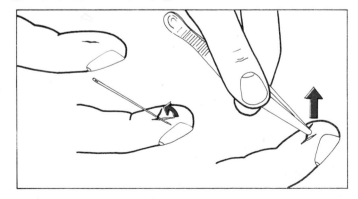

Above: Prise up the protruding end of a splinter with a sterilized needle and then gently pull it out with a pair of tweezers.

out in time, and therefore it is best to leave them alone.

3 A large or painful splinter that you cannot remove, or ANY glass or metal splinter, should be removed by a doctor.

SPRAINS & STRAINS

Muscles can sometimes be strained by over-stretching. If you have an aching back after a day's gardening it is probably because you have strained a muscle. A strain produces a sudden sharp pain and sometimes a little swelling and tenderness if you feel the spot but you can usually move the injured part quite normally, although it may be painful.

For muscular strains, no real first aid treatment is needed except rest and perhaps a hot bath.

A sprain is an injury to a joint. Sprains are more serious, more painful and take longer to heal. A joint has to be able to move, but also must be firm and stable. Strong bands of tissue, called ligaments, keep the bones firmly in place but allow the necessary movement. If you twist or wrench the joint in the 'wrong' direction – as happens when you 'go over' on an ankle on an uneven pavement, for example – you may stretch the ligament or tear it partially loose. Sometimes the ligament may be torn completely away from the bone or even tear away a small part of the bone to which it is attached. It may be impossible, without an x-ray, to tell whether you have fractured a bone or sprained a ligament but, as the initial treatment in either case is the same (except for a bad break), there is no need to rush to hospital for an x-ray straight away. Wait for a day or two to see whether the injury is getting better.

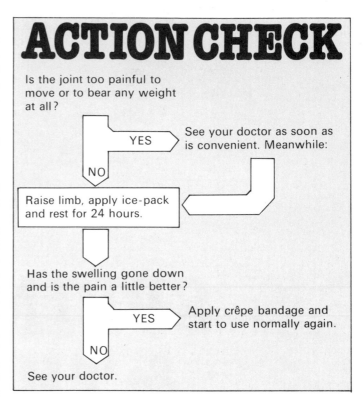

ACTION CHECK

Is the joint too painful to move or to bear any weight at all?

YES → See your doctor as soon as is convenient. Meanwhile:

NO ↓

Raise limb, apply ice-pack and rest for 24 hours.

↓

Has the swelling gone down and is the pain a little better?

YES → Apply crêpe bandage and start to use normally again.

NO ↓

See your doctor.

SYMPTOMS OF A SPRAINED JOINT

Pain, which is worse when you try to move the joint. Swelling around the joint, and later, bruising.

1 Raise the injured part and apply an ice-pack or cold compress. This helps to minimize the swelling and also relieves the pain. The most efficient ice-pack is a polythene bag filled with crushed ice and salt, but failing this, a wad of cotton wool soaked in cold, preferably iced, water and bandaged around the joint will do. Carry on the ice-pack treatment for at least half an hour. If ice or water are unavailable, apply pressure to the joint by wrapping it in a thick layer of cotton wool and bandage firmly.

2 Put on a crêpe bandage to support the joint. If a knee or ankle has been injured, use a special elasticated knee or ankle bandage.

3 Rest the joint as much as you can for the next 24 hours, keeping it raised. If you have sprained a wrist, keep the injured arm in a sling with the hand higher than the elbow.

4 After 48 hours of this treatment, the pain and swelling should have subsided. If you have sprained a knee or ankle you should be able to put a little weight on it without too much pain. If the ankle is still just as painful, or you cannot bear to put much weight on it, you should see your doctor who may suggest that you have it x-rayed. A minor sprain should be back to normal in ten days, although a bad sprain may take up to two months to heal completely. Try to use the joint as much as you can but be guided by the pain – if it hurts a lot, stop. If you sprain an ankle when you are out of doors, perhaps some way from any transport, try to improvise a bandage to give some support. Loosen any boot or shoe laces (because later swelling will make it difficult to get the shoe off) but don't remove the shoe. Bandage over it and around the ankle. Hobbling on the ankle may be painful but it won't make the injury worse.

SUNBURN

Moderate exposure to the sun will tan the skin because it stimulates the formation of the pigment melanin. Besides making the skin darker, exposure to the sun will also thicken it, and it is this thickening as much as the pigmentation that protects against burning. Too much sun-tanning will prematurely age the skin, making it permanently thick and wrinkled. The sun, like any other form of heat, will burn, and this happens if the skin is exposed to its rays for too long before some protection has been built up. The skin reddens, and then blisters. In severe cases the patient may become feverish, suffer from heatstroke, or even develop SHOCK (p. 69) as with any other severe burn.

A mildly burned skin will feel hot and itchy and if the skin becomes badly burnt it will blister. Do not prick the blisters; this will simply leave the raw skin underneath open to infection. Calamine lotion is a soothing remedy for sunburn but immersing the burnt part in cold water helps too. If you are badly burnt and blistered, feel ill or have a raised temperature, consult a doctor.

Below: Make sure your children's skin has some protection from the sun during the first days of your holiday.

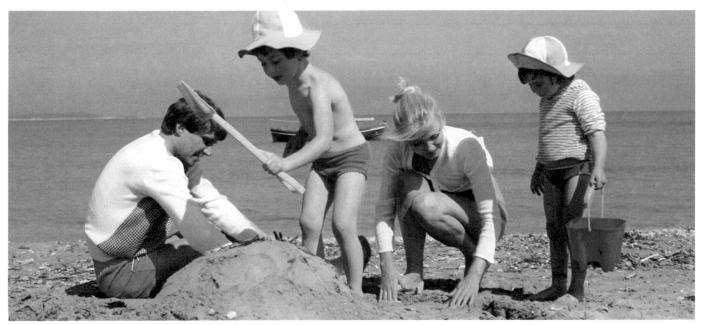

SWALLOWED OBJECTS

If your child swallows something that slips down easily you need not worry but to reassure yourself, watch his bowel movements for its reappearance within the next 24 hours. A child who has swallowed a dangerously sharp object such as an open safety pin will probably be in considerable pain. Take him to the nearest casualty department straight away. It may pass through the gut naturally but, if there is a risk of damage to the stomach or intestines, an operation may be needed.

Small pieces of bone, or fishbones, are easily swallowed accidentally and may scratch the lining of the throat or become jammed across it. Even a scratch may feel as though the bone is still stuck. If you are sure the bone is still wedged in the throat, go to the casualty department. If you are not sure, eat a piece of bread which may act as a 'wrap' for the bone and wait a few hours. If the throat is still painful, go to your doctor or hospital casualty department.

WHAT TO DO IN AN

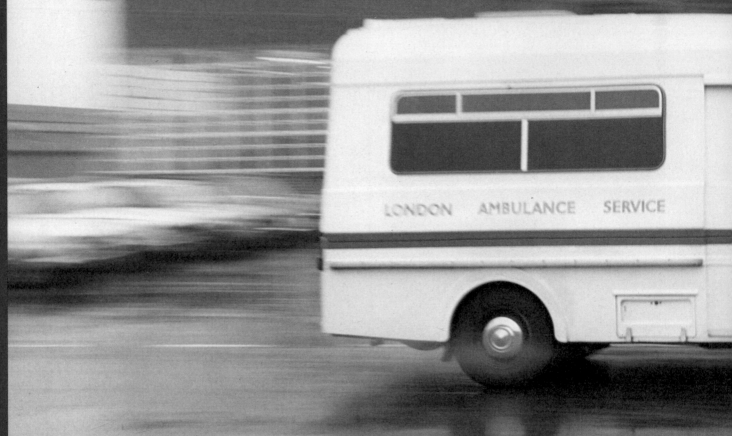

Most of the first aid measures in this book describe how to deal with everyday minor accidents since these are the situations most of us are likely to encounter. We are not, fortunately, often called upon to save lives, but there are times when knowing what to do in an emergency really is a matter of life and death. Many road-accident victims, for example, do not die from their injuries but because they have choked to death while lying unconscious. Rather horrifyingly it is estimated that a considerable number of road accident fatalities could have been saved if someone had just turned the injured person over into the recovery position described on p. 72. This section describes how to save lives: how to give artificial respiration to someone who is no longer breathing, how to give cardiac massage to someone whose heart has stopped beating. The trouble is, of course, that the times when we are likely to be faced with this sort of emergency are the moments when we are unlikely to have a first aid book neatly tucked away in our pockets. Even if we had, there would be no time to read it, for in any emergency speed is essential. If you have to consult the book before you can act you will probably be too late to save a life, so

learn the techniques before you ever need to use them. While it is quite possible to grasp the principles and basic outlines of all these methods from a book, the best way of all to learn is to attend a first aid course, so that you can watch an expert demonstrate life-saving techniques, and be taught by someone who can watch your own performance critically and show you how to improve it. This particularly applies to emergency resuscitation.

1 Make sure no one else gets hurt. An accident that initially involved only a couple of cars, for example, can easily become a motorway pile-up. The first helpers on the scene should warn or stop approaching motorists. If any 'hazard triangles' are available, place them in the roadway, or park any available cars with headlights on full beam and hazard lights flashing as a warning.

2 Summon help. 999 calls are *free*. Whoever makes the call should give as many details about the accident as possible – how many people are involved, their approximate ages and whether they are badly hurt. If it looks as though cutting or lifting gear may be needed to rescue anyone

EMERGENCY

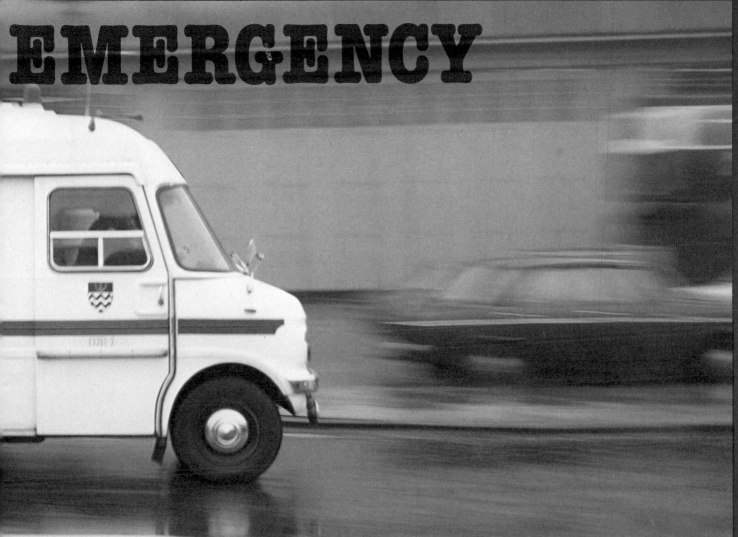

who is trapped in wreckage, this should be mentioned too.

3 Deal with the obvious emergencies first – people who are not breathing will need to be given artificial respiration (p. 70), those who are unconscious should be placed in the recovery position (p. 72) and those who are severely bleeding or burnt will need to be given the appropriate first aid treatment (p. 36 and p. 42).

4 Don't make matters worse. Move the seriously injured as little as possible unless you *have* to move them to get them out of the way of further danger – if the roof of a building looks as though it is about to cave in, for example, or if you need to place someone in the recovery position.

5 Don't give anyone who is badly injured anything to eat or drink. He may become unconscious, or need to be given a general anaesthetic if he has to be operated on. In either case, if there is anything in his stomach there is a risk that he might vomit and choke.

There are two exceptions to this rule: if some-one has swallowed a corrosive poison you should give him fluid to dilute it (see p. 62).

If someone has been badly burnt you may give him small sips of water to drink. NEVER give alcohol to anyone who has been injured or is in a state of shock.

6 Make the injured as comfortable as you can. Keep them warm but don't overheat them. A blanket *under* the body will give more protection to someone lying on cold ground than one over it. Anyone who is conscious and has no neck or back injuries can be gently moved into whatever position is most comfortable.

7 *Reassure the injured*. Perhaps this is the most difficult thing of all. It helps if *you* can manage to look – and sound – calm and in control of the situation, however panic-stricken you may feel. Don't leave them alone except very briefly, if you have to. Don't forget that an apparently unconscious casualty may be able to overhear what is being said around him. If any people are standing aimlessly by, take command of the situation and tell them what you want them to do to help you.

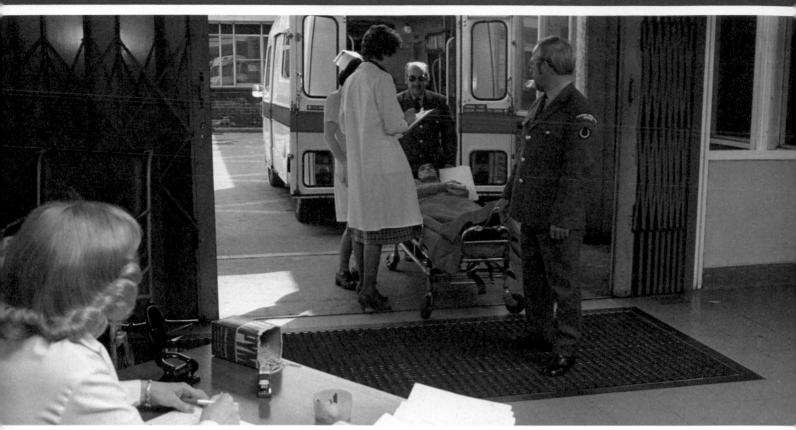

THE HOSPITAL CASUALTY DEPARTMENT

After a severe accident, the casualty will be taken by ambulance to the nearest hospital casualty department. If you are involved in a minor accident, a friend or relative may drive you to the hospital, but REMEMBER there are only one or two accident departments in each district.

What will happen on your arrival at the casualty department:

1 The casualty sister will assess your condition and decide whether you need immediate emergency treatment or whether you can take your turn with the other patients. She will also decide whether you are a medical or surgical emergency.

2 If you are conscious you will be asked to give your name, address, religion and next of kin. This is just routine procedure, and does not mean that anything awful is expected to happen to you.

3 If possible, go armed with a good book, for unless you are a real emergency, or very lucky, you may well have to wait a long time before you are examined by a doctor. When your turn comes, the doctor will ask for details of your accident, and may send you for further tests or investigations. X-rays may also be needed, particularly if you have broken a bone. Any cuts will be stitched in the casualty department.

Above: The Casualty Department is the hospital's 'Clearing House'. Here your condition will be assessed and you will be given whatever immediate treatment is needed before being discharged or transferred to another department.

If you have had a suspected heart attack, you will be given an *electrocardiogram*. This measures the electrical activity of the heart muscle which is altered in disease and will entail electrodes being attached to your arms, legs and chest. Although it may seem rather alarming, it is completely painless, and will help the doctor to check whether your heart is functioning normally.

4 If your injuries are severe; if you have had a suspected heart attack or are brought in unconscious, you will be admitted to the hospital. If you are unconscious, the hospital staff will search your pockets to discover your identity. If you do not have a friend or relative with you, the hospital will advise the police, who will contact your next of kin – provided they know who you are. So make sure that you always carry some form of identification with you.

5 You may regain consciousness after a serious accident and find yourself in the hospital *intensive care unit*. Here you will probably be nursed on a bed in an open space, surrounded by electronic monitoring equipment.

SHOCK

Shock is the term used to describe the symptoms that arise when the body organs, especially the brain, are deprived of blood. What we usually think of as shock – the feeling of faintness or shakiness that can follow a slight injury or an emotional upset – is caused by a temporary loss of blood to the brain, see FAINTING (p. 55) and is not life-threatening. True, medical shock occurs when there is actually less blood or body fluid available. When this happens, the body tries to keep up the blood supply to the brain at the expense of all other, less important parts of the body.

Body fluid may be lost by:

● Severe bleeding, either internal or external.

● Loss of plasma from burns, scalds or crush injuries.

● Loss of output by the heart following a serious heart attack.

● Loss of body fluid due to persistent vomiting or diarrhoea.

● An abdominal emergency such as a perforated stomach ulcer or a burst appendix.

An adult can lose up to one pint of body fluid (the amount taken if you become a blood donor) without any effect except a slightly increased pulse-rate. As more fluid is lost, the heart beats faster still, in an effort to keep up the supply, but because there is less blood to pump, the blood pressure falls and the casualty will feel faint or shaky. Blood is shunted away first from the skin, which becomes pale, cold and clammy, and then from the muscles, so that he becomes weak. As more fluid is lost, the brain itself will become deprived of blood so that he becomes confused, agitated and eventually unconscious. Unless medical help is given, and the lost fluid is replaced with blood or plasma transfusion, shock will lead to failure of breathing and of the heart.

After a severe accident always watch for the signs of shock:

● Cold, clammy skin with heavy sweating
● Faintness, giddiness or blurring of vision
● Nausea or vomiting
● Thirst
● Confusion and anxiety
● Rapid, shallow breathing
● Rapid, feeble pulse.

1 Lie the casualty down with his feet raised, and his head turned to one side.

2 Deal with the cause of shock if this is possible – by stopping heavy bleeding for example.

3 Send for help. You must get him into hospital as soon as you can.

4 Do not move him unnecessarily. If he is unconscious or seems likely to vomit, place him in the RECOVERY POSITION (p. 72).

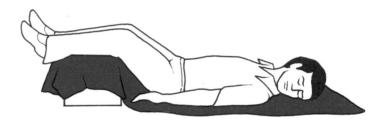

Above: Providing he is conscious and breathing normally a patient suffering from shock should be placed on his back, with his head turned to one side and his legs raised. If possible, lie him on a blanket or coat.

5 If his head, chest or stomach are injured, raise his head and shoulders slightly and support them.

6 Loosen any tight clothing.

7 Stop further heat loss. Put a blanket *under* him. Cover him if he shivers, but *do not* use hot-water bottles or electric blankets – this only draws blood back to the skin, which does not need it, away from the vital body organs, which do.

8 DO NOT GIVE ANYTHING (especially not alcohol) to drink, but moisten his lips with water if he is thirsty.

OLD WIVES' TALE

It is not true that there is nothing so good as a glass of brandy for anyone who is shocked. Alcohol will in fact make the condition *worse*, by opening up small blood vessels in the skin so that more blood flows through them – at the expense of the brain and other important organs in the body.

ARTIFICIAL RESPIRATION

The unconscious person who is NOT BREATHING is being starved of oxygen. If the brain is deprived of oxygen for more than four minutes it will probably be permanently damaged. Your first priority is to keep up an emergency supply of air to his lungs. The simplest and most effective way of doing this is by breathing into the lungs yourself. The air that you breathe out will not be as oxygen-rich as the air the casualty would normally breathe in, but it will be quite adequate to maintain life and avoid brain-damage. This method is called MOUTH-TO-MOUTH RESUSCITATION or EXPIRED AIR RESUSCITATION, and it is suitable in nearly all cases. You may need to use another method if there is severe facial injury, or if the casualty is pinned face downwards so that you cannot turn him, or if he begins to vomit.

MOUTH-TO-MOUTH
START TO RESUSCITATE IMMEDIATELY.

1 DO NOT waste time in fetching help or dealing with any other injury. If you *think* the casualty is not breathing, artificial respiration will do no harm, so don't spend vital moments making sure.

2 Put his head well back (you should be looking down into his nostrils), and pull his jaw forward. This brings the tongue forward clear of the airway and may be enough in itself to start him breathing again. Loosen tight clothing at his neck.

3 With a finger, dig into his mouth to make sure that no foreign matter or vomit is blocking the airway. If he has *loose* false teeth, remove them. Otherwise, leave them in place – they help to keep the mouth in shape and make artificial respiration easier.

4 Pinch his nostrils together, otherwise the air will take the easiest way out, and make sure that his mouth is open.

5 Take a deep breath and put your mouth over his, making as good a seal as you can with your lips. Blow into his lungs four times, blowing from your chest rather than your cheeks, as quickly as you can. Watch his chest each time – it should rise as the air enters his lungs. If it does not, and if his head is tilted well back, there must be some obstruction. Turn him on to one side and slap him smartly on the back, between the shoulder blades. Check again with a finger to see if any foreign matter is blocking the back of his throat.

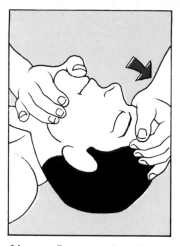
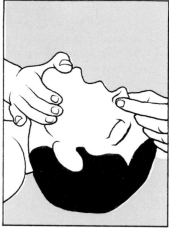

Above: Ensure a clear airway by tilting the head back and the jaw forward. Hold the mouth open and pinch nostrils shut.

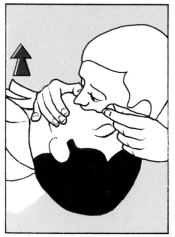
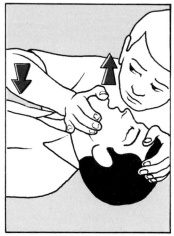

Above: Breathe into his mouth and watch his chest rise. As you take your mouth away his chest should fall.

6 Carry on breathing into his lungs. You will find it difficult to keep up your normal breathing rate (which is about 15–18 breaths per minute). Find a steady, comfortable pace which you can keep up easily. If you blow too quickly you will make yourself feel faint. Don't blow too hard – just hard enough to make the chest rise. Don't be discouraged if he does not start to breathe straight away. There are cases of people who have been revived after as long as 8 hours of artificial respiration. Keep it up until he starts to breathe again or until expert help arrives.

7 As soon as he does start to breathe again, place him in the RECOVERY POSITION (p. 72).

SMALL CHILDREN

If the casualty is an infant or a small child, seal your mouth around his mouth and nose together. Blow *gently* into his lungs until his chest rises, and then continue as for an adult (see above).

MOUTH-TO-NOSE

If you cannot open the casualty's mouth, or if it is badly injured, you may be able to use mouth-to-nose resuscitation. The principle is the same as mouth-to-mouth resuscitation, but you should breathe through the casualty's *nose*, keeping one hand beneath his chin so that his mouth is kept closed, as shown below.

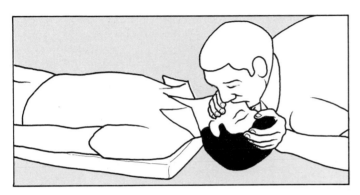

ALTERNATIVE METHODS OF ARTIFICIAL RESPIRATION

Mouth-to-mouth (or mouth-to-nose) resuscitation is *always* the best method to use if it can be done. But there are times when it is not practicable either because the casualty's face is too badly injured or because he is trapped in a position that makes it impossible.

In these circumstances there are two alternative methods that can be used, both of which are techniques for physically expanding and contracting the chest so that air is drawn into and expelled from the lungs. The Holger-Nielsen method is the best of the two in cases of drowning, as the casualty is face down so that fluid can easily drain from his lungs, and it may be the only choice if he happens to be pinned face downwards so that you cannot turn him over. The Sylvester method has the advantage that you can use external cardiac massage as well, if necessary (p. 74), so it is the method of choice in a non-breathing casualty whose heart has also stopped.

THE HOLGER-NIELSEN METHOD

1 Place the casualty face downwards, his head turned to one side and pillowed on his hands. Kneel on one knee at his head, placing your other foot near his elbow. Put your hands on his back just below the shoulder blades and touching each other.

2 With your elbows straight, rock forward so that the pressure forces the air from his lungs.

3 Grasp the casualty's elbows.

4 Rock backwards so that his arms are brought forward and raised. This expands his chest and draws air into the lungs.

Repeat this whole manoeuvre, trying to set up a steady rate without pausing between the two parts of the cycle – each half of the cycle should take about 2½ seconds. As soon as the casualty starts to breathe naturally, place him in the RECOVERY POSITION (p. 72).

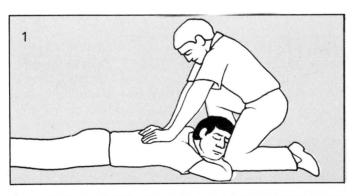

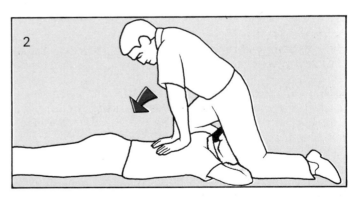

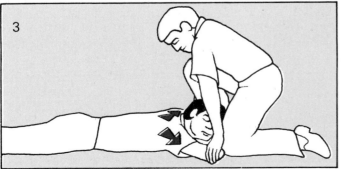

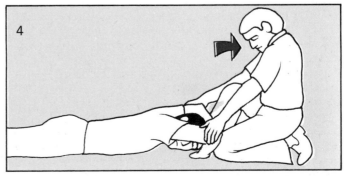

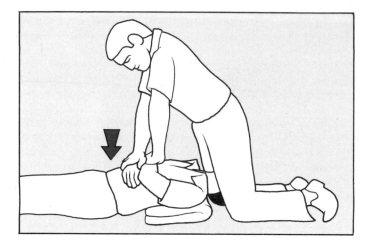

Above: Drive the air from the patient's chest by rocking forward with your weight on his crossed arms.

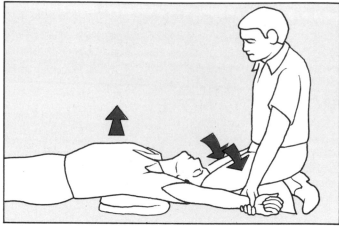

Above: Sweep his arms up, out and back as far as you can so that they are spreadeagled on either side of his head.

THE SYLVESTER METHOD:

1 Lie the unconscious person on his back on a firm surface, and put a folded jacket or blanket beneath his shoulders so that they are slightly raised. His head should be tipped backwards.

2 Sweep a finger around inside his mouth to make sure nothing is blocking his airway.

3 Kneel behind him so that his head is between your knees. Take his wrists and cross them over the lower part of his chest.

4 With your arms straight, rock forwards so that the weight of your body drives the air from his lungs.

5 Rock backwards, sweeping his arms backwards and outwards as far as you can. This movement expands the rib cage so that air is drawn into the lungs.

6 Try to carry out this whole manoeuvre at as near a normal breathing rate as you can manage – about 12 times a minute.

UNCONSCIOUSNESS

Unconsciousness can be caused by anything that interrupts the normal working of the brain, or reduces the circulation of blood to the brain. The most common causes, for example suffocation, shock, heart attack, head injuries, poisoning, epilepsy and diabetic emergency, are dealt with elsewhere.

Whatever has caused the patient's unconsciousness may also have caused additional injuries. His breathing may have stopped, for example, or he may be bleeding severely. Your first priority is to deal with any of these life-threatening injuries. Once this has been done you can take steps to prevent the main threat to the unconscious patient, which is that he may choke to death. He may vomit and will be unable to cough or gag to prevent the vomit getting into his lungs, or his tongue may fall limply to the back of his throat, obstructing his airway so that he cannot breathe. These dangers can be eliminated simply by turning him on to his side into the RECOVERY POSITION. You should NOT move any unconscious person who has had a bad fall or serious injury which may have damaged his spine. LEAVE HIM WHERE HE IS until help arrives.

THE RECOVERY POSITION

● Before you try to turn the person, loosen any tight clothing around his neck, check that he is breathing and that his airway is clear, remove glasses if he is wearing them and remove, too, any loose false teeth.

● Kneel beside him on his left hand side, and tuck the hand nearest to you well underneath his bottom, keeping the arm and the fingers as straight as possible.

● Cross the arm furthest from you over his chest, and the leg furthest from you over the nearer leg.

● Grasp his clothing at the hip and roll him over on to your lap. Keep your right hand under his cheek as you turn him, to protect his head.

● Draw his top knee up so that it forms a right angle with his body, then move away from him. Draw his top arm up to make a right angle with his body, and bend it at the elbow. If the ground is rough, cushion his face on this hand.

● Make sure that his head is turned to one side, tilted well back with the chin pushed forwards.

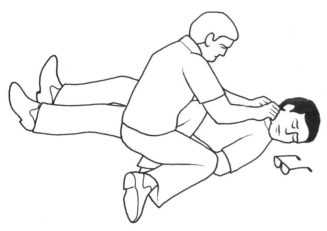

1. Loosen tight clothing and remove glasses before placing the patient in the recovery position.

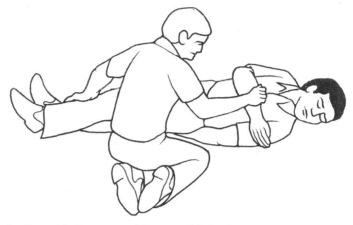

2. Cross his far arm and leg over his body.

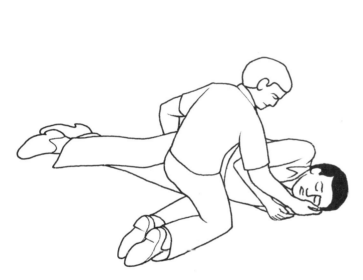

3. Cradling his head in your hand, pull his hip sharply up and over.

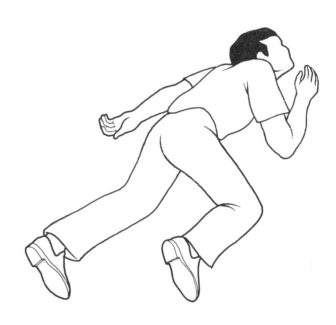

4. Bend his top arm and leg at a right angle and tilt his head back so that his chin juts forward.

DEALING WITH THE UNCONSCIOUS PATIENT

1 Make sure that the casualty's airway is clear, by sweeping a finger wrapped in a handkerchief around inside his mouth.

2 Check that he is breathing. If he is not, start ARTIFICIAL RESPIRATION (p. 70).

3 Deal with any serious BLEEDING (p. 36).

4 Place him in the RECOVERY POSITION (see above). If you feel that he is too badly injured to risk moving, turn his head to one side, pushing his jaw forwards.

5 Summon a doctor or ambulance as quickly as you can.

6 Look to see if he is carrying a Medic-Alert card or bracelet. This could indicate that he is a DIABETIC (p. 52) or an EPILEPTIC (p. 49). If you find lumps of sugar in his pocket, this suggests that he may be a diabetic.

7 Cover him with a blanket and if possible place one under him as well.

8 Stay with him until help arrives.

9 Don't try to give him anything to drink. If he recovers consciousness, and is thirsty, you can moisten his lips with water.

EXTERNAL
CARDIAC MASSAGE

The heart lies just behind the lower end of the breast-bone. If it has stopped beating it is sometimes possible to stimulate the heart muscle to contract by pressing the breast-bone down so that it squeezes the heart, forcing blood into the circulation. Many first aid manuals do not mention cardiac massage, because this is strictly a job for the experts. The very good reason for this is that it is difficult to tell whether the heart *has* stopped beating, and if cardiac massage is carried out on a heart which *is* still beating, even very weakly, there is a danger that the heartbeat may become dangerously irregular and perhaps stop altogether. But the technique can be life-saving and should be learned properly at first aid classes (p. 78). In an emergency, where no other help is available, and where you are CERTAIN that the heart has stopped beating, you can follow the instructions below.

HOW TO TELL IF THE HEART IS NOT BEATING

1 Feel the casualty's pulse. The carotid pulse, in the neck, is always stronger than the pulse at the wrist, so this is the best place to feel it. (Practise on yourself, by placing your fingers and thumb on either side of the neck, below the jaw, until you can feel the pulse easily.) If you are still in any doubt, put your ear to the casualty's chest, slightly to the left of the lower end of the breast-bone. If there is any heart-beat, you should be able to hear it.

IF THE HEART HAS STOPPED THERE WILL BE NO PULSE.

2 Look at his colour.

IF THE HEART HAS STOPPED THE CASUALTY'S FACE WILL BE EXTREMELY PALE OR BLUE-GREY AND BLUE AROUND THE LIPS.

3 Raise his eyelids and look at his pupils.

IF THE HEART HAS STOPPED HIS PUPILS WILL BE VERY ENLARGED.

REMEMBER
If you can feel the pulse, even if it is very weak, DO NOT start cardiac massage.

The heart action is the last of the body's vital functions to stop. So anyone whose heart is not beating will not be breathing either. Cardiac massage to start the heart has to be combined with mouth-to-mouth resuscitation to maintain an air supply to the lungs. Even after the heart has started beating, you will probably need to carry on mouth-to-mouth resuscitation for a little while longer until the casualty starts breathing naturally again.

1 Lie the casualty on a hard surface. If you are dealing with, for example, a heart-attack patient who is in bed you must try to get him on to the floor. You cannot carry out cardiac massage on a springy mattress.

2 Make sure that his airway is clear, by tilting the head backwards and pulling the jaw forwards. Quickly sweep around inside the mouth with a finger if there is a chance that any foreign matter might be obstructing the airway.

3 Give four quick mouth-to-mouth breaths, pinching his nostrils together and sealing your own lips around his mouth.

4 Feel the carotid pulse.

5 If you can still feel no pulse, thump once, either with the side of your hand or with a clenched fist, slightly to the left of the lower part of the breast-bone, about one handspan down from the top of the collar-bone. 'Bounce' your fist off the ribs – don't let it go dead on them. This may be enough to start the heart beating again.

6 Feel the carotid pulse once more. If you can feel it, carry on doing mouth-to-mouth resuscitation until he starts to breathe naturally again.

7 If there is still no pulse, place the heel of one of your hands on the lower part of the breast-bone, keeping your thumb and fingers off the chest, and cover this with the heel of your other hand. Then rock forwards with your arms straight so that you push the breast-bone down about 4 cm ($1\frac{1}{2}$ in). (An easy way to practise this is to use a pair of bathroom scales – you need to exert a pressure on the scales of about 5–6 kg (12–14 lb).) If you are reviving a child use only one hand's pressure, and for a baby, the pressure of two fingers is enough. Give one compression per second for an adult, but use a slightly quicker rate for children and a considerably quicker one for infants (aim for 100 compressions per minute).

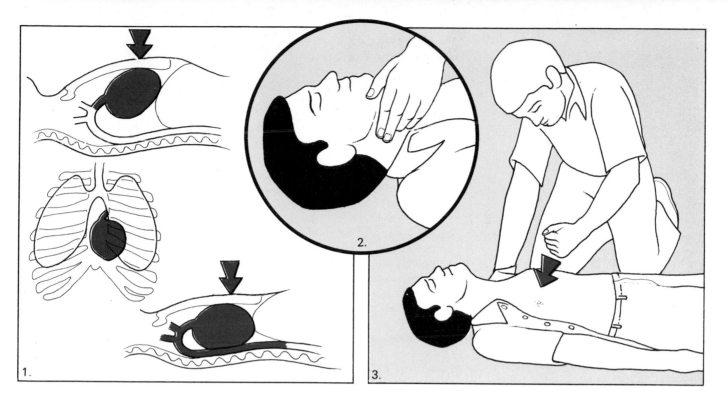

1. Cross-section of the chest showing how pressure applied with the heels of the hands 'squeezes' the heart between the breast-bone and the spine.

2. Check the carotid pulse.

3. If you cannot feel any pulse, striking the chest to the left of the lower part of the breastbone may be enough to start the heart beating.

8 After each FIVE compressions, give one mouth-to-mouth breath. Then check the carotid pulse once more. Try to be firm but not violent in your pressure or you may damage internal organs or break ribs.

9 Repeat this sequence until you can see that you have been successful because:

● You are able to feel the carotid pulse

● You can see that his colour is improving

● You can see that his pupils have returned to their normal size.

When this happens, carry on giving mouth-to-mouth resuscitation until he starts to breathe once more.

10 Turn him over into the RECOVERY POSITION (p. 72).

If someone is available to help you the process is easier. One of you should give cardiac massage, the other should give mouth-to-mouth resuscitation and be responsible for checking the pulse. But keep to the same rhythm – one breath, followed by five cardiac compressions.

DON'T
Don't try to give cardiac massage and mouth-to-mouth resuscitation simultaneously. Even if you have a helper, always alternate the two procedures.

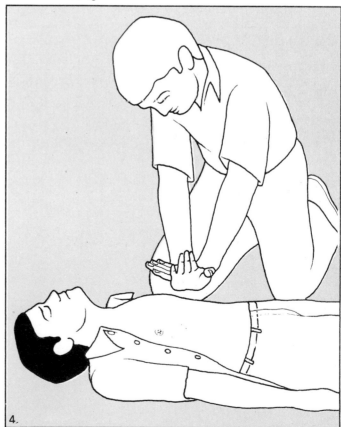

4. If there is still no pulse, apply pressure with the heels of your hands on the lower part of the breastbone to 'squeeze' the heart and force blood around the body.

GLOSSARY

AFTERBIRTH (placenta)
The structure on the wall of the uterus to which the fetus is attached by the umbilical cord. It provides nourishment for the baby in the womb and is normally expelled a few minutes after the baby's birth.

ALLERGY
The body's hypersensitive reaction to a foreign substance. Allergic reactions usually affect the skin, causing a rash and itching, or the respiratory system, for example the runny nose and watery eyes of hay fever, or the wheezy breathing of asthma.

ANALGESIC
A pain-killing drug such as aspirin or paracetamol.

ANGINA PECTORIS
A sudden constricting pain in the chest usually radiating to one or both shoulders and arms. It is brought on by physical exertion because the heart muscle is temporarily deprived of oxygen.

ANTI-HISTAMINE
A drug which is commonly used in treating allergic reactions like hay fever.

ANTISEPTIC
A chemical that kills germs and inhibits their growth. It may also damage body cells if used in too strong a solution.

ARTERY
A blood vessel carrying blood away from the heart.

ARTIFICIAL RESPIRATION
Any method for artificially 'pumping' air into and out of the lungs when natural breathing has stopped.

ASPHYXIA
Suffocation caused when the oxygen supply of the body is cut off so that air cannot pass in or out of the lungs.

ASPIRIN
A drug commonly used to relieve pain and to lower a raised temperature.

ASTHMA
A condition which comes on suddenly when there is severe difficulty in breathing with a feeling of constriction and suffocation. It can often be attributed to an allergic condition.

ATHEROMA
A fatty material which is sometimes deposited in the lining of arteries so that they become narrowed.

BACTERIA
Microscopic, single-celled organisms, some of which can cause disease.

BLISTER
A fluid-filled 'bubble' in the skin, usually caused by rubbing or by burning. Blood blisters may form if the skin is sharply pinched.

BRUISE
Discoloration of the skin caused by bleeding into the tissues beneath it.

CALAMINE LOTION
A soothing, slightly astringent lotion which is often used for treating sunburn or minor skin irritations.

CARDIAC MASSAGE
See HEART MASSAGE.

COLD COMPRESS
A soft pad of absorbent fabric which is soaked in cold water. The excess water is squeezed out and the compress is applied to a bruise or swelling to help reduce pain and swelling.

COMA
See UNCONSCIOUSNESS.

COMPRESSION (OF THE BRAIN)
Pressure on the brain is usually caused either by a depressed bone from a fractured skull, or by blood which has leaked from a broken blood vessel inside the skull. The patient may become drowsy, confused and then gradually lapses into unconsciousness.

CONCUSSION
A short period of unconsciousness or impaired consciousness following a head injury, caused by a 'shaking up' of the brain inside the skull.

CONSCIOUSNESS
The state of being awake, alert and aware of what is going on around you.

CONTRACTION (in childbirth)
'Labour pains' — the rhythmical shortening and relaxation of the muscles of the womb that gradually open up the birth canal and propel the baby through it.

CONVULSION
A violent involuntary muscular contraction due to a disturbance of brain function.

CORONARY ARTERY DISEASE
A disease in which the walls of the arteries that supply blood to the heart become thickened and the interior narrowed. The same general narrowing process can affect all the arteries in the body but has the most serious consequences when those arteries supplying the heart and brain are affected.

CORONARY THROMBOSIS
Another name for a 'heart attack'. A sudden complete blockage of one of the arteries that supply blood to the heart muscle. The severity of the attack depends on how much of the heart muscle is affected.

CORROSIVE LIQUID
One which burns because it is strongly acid or alkaline. If inhaled, a corrosive liquid can severely damage the lungs so especial care is needed in cases of poisoning by such liquids.

CRAMP
A sudden, painful muscle spasm.

DIABETES
A disease caused by an insufficiency of a substance called insulin, which normally controls the sugar level in the blood. Symptoms include the presence of sugar in the urine, passing of excessive amounts of urine, thirst and often loss of weight.

DIRECT PRESSURE
A method of stopping bleeding by applying direct pressure on the wound.

DISLOCATION
Displacement of one or more of the bones forming a joint (or of an organ) from its normal position. The ligaments that bind the joint together may be torn; this is usually caused by a severe twist or wrench.

DIZZINESS
A feeling of giddiness, sometimes caused by a temporary lack of blood to the brain.

DRUG
Any substance used as a medicine.

EPILEPSY
Recurrent episodes of abnormal electrical brain activity leading to loss of consciousness and convulsions.

FAINTING
A brief loss of consciousness, caused by diminished blood flow to the brain.

FIT
See CONVULSION.

FRACTURE
A break, usually of bone.
TYPES OF FRACTURE
CLOSED A fracture of bone in which the skin surface is not broken.
COMPLICATED A fracture in which the broken bone has damaged some important adjacent body structure, such as the lungs or liver.
GREENSTICK An incomplete fracture affecting the young, pliable bones of children. The bone bends or cracks like a green twig, but does not break completely.
OPEN A fracture in which there is an open wound through which infection can reach the broken bone.

GERM
The term applied to any microscopic organism which can cause disease.

HEART ATTACK
See CORONARY THROMBOSIS.

HEART COMPRESSION (EXTERNAL)
See HEART MASSAGE.

HEART MASSAGE (EXTERNAL)
A method which should only be used by a qualified first-aider for re-starting the heart after it has stopped beating.

HEAT EXHAUSTION
A condition brought on by loss of salt and water from the body. This often occurs in very hot climates or conditions.

HEATSTROKE
A condition characterised by a rapidly developing high temperature and severe prostration, caused by the body's inability to lose enough heat in very hot or humid conditions.

HEIMLICH MANOEUVRE
A technique for shooting out an obstruction in the throat by giving the abdomen a sudden, violent squeeze.

HOLGER-NIELSEN
A method of artificial respiration which can be used when the face is injured and mouth-to-mouth resuscitation is not practicable. By manipulating the patient's body and arms air is forced in and out of the lungs.

HYPOTHERMIA
Lowering of the body temperature to 35°C (95°F) or less, caused by exposure to cold, wet or windy conditions.

IMMOBILIZATION OF FRACTURES
Supporting a broken limb so that the fractured bones cannot be moved, either by use of a splint (metal, wood, plastic, rolled-up magazines or newspapers) or an adjacent part of the casualty's body as a means of support.

KAOLIN
A chalk-like powder which, given in solution, is used to treat stomach upsets.

KISS OF LIFE
See MOUTH-TO-MOUTH RESUSCITATION.

LABOUR
The process of giving birth. Labour is divided into three stages — the first being the opening up of the birth canal, the second the actual birth of the baby, and the third the expulsion of the afterbirth or placenta.

LIGAMENT
A tough, fibrous band connecting one bone to another.

MISCARRIAGE (spontaneous abortion)
The expulsion of a fetus before the 28th week of pregnancy.

MOUTH-TO-MOUTH RESUSCITATION
A method of artificial respiration in which the rescuer breathes air from his own lungs into the casualty's lungs, through the casualty's mouth or nose.

PARACETAMOL
A drug commonly used to relieve pain and to lower a raised temperature.

PRESSURE POINTS
These are points at which an artery passes over a bone, and can be pressed against it to stop severe bleeding. The two pressure points most easily found by first-aiders are the BRACHIAL PRESSURE POINT on the inside of the upper arm, and the FEMORAL PRESSURE POINT at the centre of the fold of the groin.

PULSE
The rhythmic throbbing which can be felt in an artery as the blood is propelled along it. Each throb corresponds to each beat of the heart. The pulse can most easily be felt on the inside of the wrist. The CAROTID PULSE is felt in the neck, on either side of the jaw and just below it.

RABIES
A viral disease of the nervous system in which the sufferer dies in agony from paralysis and convulsions. If a course of anti-rabies injections is given promptly, before the first symptoms appear, the disease can be prevented.

RECOVERY POSITION
The position into which all unconscious patients should be put (except those with a suspected spinal injury). The patient is placed lying on one side, his head tilted slightly backwards and his top arm and leg bent at a right-angle to support him. The recovery position prevents the casualty from choking and allows fluids to drain from the mouth.

RESUSCITATION
The restoration of either heart-beat or breathing.

SHOCK
A state of collapse which may follow any serious injury and is due to a reduction in the volume of circulating fluid in the body.

SPINAL COLUMN
The backbone of the body, through which the SPINAL CORD runs. The spinal cord is the delicate nerve trunk leading from the brain to the base of the spine and any fracture of the spinal column involves the risk of damaging nerves and causing loss of feeling or movement in some part of the body.

SPRAIN
An injury in which the ligaments binding the bones in a joint together are torn or stretched, but the bones themselves are not displaced.

STRAIN
A minor muscle injury in which the muscle fibres are over-stretched. Usually caused by sudden severe exertion.

STROKE (cerebral haemorrhage or cerebrovascular accident)
Damage to the brain caused by the clotting or bursting of a blood vessel within it. The results of a stroke can vary from a temporary loss of functioning of one part of the body to major paralysis, unconsciousness or death.

SYLVESTER METHOD
A method of artificial respiration which is sometimes used when facial injuries make mouth-to-mouth resuscitation impracticable. By manipulating the casualty's arms and chest, air is drawn into and expelled from his lungs.

TEMPERATURE
The normal temperature of the healthy human body is 37°C (98.4°F) though it may be slightly lower first thing in the morning and slightly higher in the evening. A rise in body temperature (or fever) is usually a sign of an infectious illness.

TENDON
A bundle of tough, stringy fibres connecting a muscle to a bone.

TETANUS
An infectious disease that causes muscle spasm and damage to the heart. The germs that cause the disease are found in earth or places that may be contaminated by animal dung, such as farmyards or parks. There is always a risk that a dirty wound or animal bite may be infected with tetanus germs, so an anti-tetanus injection is usually given as a guard against infection.

UNCONSCIOUSNESS
A state of insensibility in which the casualty does not respond to stimuli.

VEIN
A blood vessel carrying blood to the heart.

FIRST AID COURSES

The British Red Cross Society offers training courses in First Aid, Occupational First Aid, Safety, Accident Prevention, Fire Prevention and Survival and Nursing to people of all age groups, from five years upwards. Special Courses may also be designed to meet special needs. Further information may be obtained from your local Branch Headquarters of the British Red Cross Society. The address and telephone number will be in the telephone directory.

INDEX

ACKNOWLEDGEMENTS

Ardea 34, 35; Art
Directors Photo Library
30; Daily Telegraph
Colour Library (S. J.
Allen) 68; London
Ambulance Service 2–3;
Leo Mason 20; Scottish
Tourist Board 19, 21;
Spectrum Colour Library
13, 22; Zefa Picture
Library 23, (G. Mabbs)
66–67, (Anthea Sieveking) 65

Special Photography:
Gina Harris 1, 29, 32–33;
Sandra Lousada 7, 8–9,
14, 15, 17, 18, 31, 47.